Principles and Practices of HERBAL GARDEN

Principles and Practices of HERBAL GARDEN

B.C. Mazumdar
Paramita Mitra Mukhopadhyay

2022

Daya Publishing House®
A Division of
Astral International Pvt. Ltd.
New Delhi – 110 002

First Published, 2006
ISBN: 9788170353782 (HB)

Published by : **Daya Publishing House®**
A Division of
Astral International Pvt. Ltd.
– ISO 9001:2015 Certified Company –
4736/23, Ansari Road, Darya Ganj
New Delhi-110 002
Ph. 011-43549197, 23278134
e-mail: info@astralint.com
Website: www.astralint.com

Digitally Printed at : **Replika Press Pvt. Ltd.**

Dedicated to the venerated memory of *Bharat Ratna*

Dr. Bidhan Chandra Roy,

D.Sc., M.B., M.R.C.P., F.R.C.S.

(July 1, 1882–July 1, 1962)
who
held a high esteem on the medicinal
plants grown in the soils,
mountains and waters in our country

Preface

The importance of medicinal plants needs no emphasis in India where very poor to very rich people hold these materials in high esteem to get rid of various types of afflictions. However, although a large section of people in this country attach much tenet on use of these plants in crude form either to cure ailments or as prophylactic, well-timed availability of these materials in safe condition becomes a difficult situation many a time. Lack of organized and widespread culture of these plants coupled with lack of their identification are among other, the notable factors that stand in the way to procure materials that are genuine and free from pollutants. This practical difficulty can however, be much averted by cropping these plants under controlled condition and the task can be taken up by individuals or by institutions, schools, colleges, clubs, communities, municipalities, panchayats and such other organizations. Evidently such steps might ensure supply of these plants to the users at he opportune moment and in safe form. This concept needs establishment of plantation of these herbals, which are popularly known as Herbal Gardens.

The concerned plants exclusively being used as medicines, obviously necessitate some special measures in their culture following organic method of farming in particular, dispensing with agro-chemicals, especially those that are liable to act upon human health or produce adverse side-effects. Authentic books pertaining to the cropping methods with that perspective being not adequately available under the conditions of India, the present title has been attempted which has considered a few medicinal plants of common usage and has brought in their cultivation procedure apart from citation of medicinal properties associated with them. The title would therefore, cater to the requirements of those who are desirous to establish and maintain herbal gardens for practical purpose as well as the students and researchers of various disciplines who are concerned with the subject notably agricultural and horticultural sciences, applied botany, ayurveda, pharmaco-botany, pharmacognosy etc.

The authors gratefully acknowledge those who have extended hands to compile the present title. Of particular mention is the Narendrapur Ramakrishna Mission whose kind co-operation in taking the photographs presented in the book is expressed with gratitude. Various types of assistance received from Dr. Achintya Mitra, M.D.(Ay.), are also gratefully acknowledged.

Lastly, the authors look forward receiving valued suggestions from the readers and persons of eminence in order that the text can be suitably enriched in future.

Calcutta University **Authors**

Contents

Chapter 1

Introduction and Objectives

The enormous benefits of various plants to resist against and recover from illness of not only human beings but also animals were intuitively recognized centuries ago by the primitive people. Plants have anchored to the Mother Earth long before man has set his feet and it is said that God had endowed them with materials for survival of man and animal long before these creatures were made by him.

The plant kingdom is directly or indirectly giving us food, clothings and materials for our dwelling. But these apart, they directly render unreckonable service to us in making provision of the essentials that bring us relief from diseases. As a matter of fact, the members of the plant kingdom not only restore health to us from illness but are also mighty weapons for our defense against diseases.

The plants cover much more geographical area than what has so far been occupied by the human beings. They have found place from the ocean-floor to the mountain-peaks and from the ardour of the deserts to the ice-clapped regions of the higher latitudes in this planet. Wide multiplicity in their structural and functional features are no doubt, a great wonderment. Right from very minute or microscopic forms, these living beings exist in gigantic appearance across the world from undifferentiated shape to the highly organized body parts, which led the botanists to classify them as belonging to the lower or the higher groups.

The common saying that each and every plant seen by us having at least some medicinal value to man is perhaps not much exaggerated. Since time immemorial, man has searched plants that would relieve pain and get rid of ailments. The curative properties of plants are thought to have come to the knowledge of the ancient people through extensive searching of plants and examining their uses and many of such assays are considered not only treacherous but even led to health hazards and casualities. Through this process, the primitive man had learnt which plant could cure a disease and which was a poison that could kill a person.

The knowledge on medicinal plants has been stated to have gathered by man since 1770 B.C. in Babylon but perhaps it was known even much earlier in India. Mention may be made to the epic, Ramayana in India, which had stated existence of such plant in the *Gandhamadan* mountain that could bring back life to Lakhsmana.

The disease curing properties of many medicinal plants were known to the ancient Egyptians as early as 1500 B.C. and in Greece during 370 B.C. Interestingly, Hippocrates believed the usefulness of "botanical drugs" as curative agents of many diseases.

The exploration of plants to serve as drugs to the human beings in the pre-historic times had in fact been done in many countries of the then world and notably, Egypt, India and China, which is evident from ancient literature, tablets, mythologic stories, poems, folk-lores etc. that were available later. Undoubtedly, India was a leading country to explore medicinal properties of many plants, which is known from the *Atharva veda*, *Rig veda* and also as mentioned in the *Samhitas* of *Charaka* and *Susurta*. It is conjectured that the *soma* had perhaps the first medicinal plant used by the Aryans in India. The juice of the plant is believed to possess intoxicating and many other medicinal properties and the plant had also been known to be used by the Aryans for sacrificial purposes.

It needs commenting upon the fact that majority of the drugs that are known today under different systems of medicine across the world have their origin from various plant species. The medicinal properties of many plants have though been hitherto known, a vast majority are left that are yet to be explored.

Necessity of Herbal Gardens

It is an admitted fact that in ancient India when the ayurvedic culture was in high esteem, the mine of knowledge on the therapeutic and prophylactic properties of various plants was not only confined to the erudite ayurveda scholars but much of that had spread to the common people as well. In those days, it was a practice among them to grow some medicinal plants in their homestead land and make use of those when any member of the family was afflicted with an ordinary ailment. However, the culture on herbal drugs by the common people in this country had been on the wane perhaps since the 17th century with introduction of other systems of medicine.

The present day practice to the majority of the common people in this country is to learn about these plants from others and notably from the senior members of the family. The trend is hardly supportable as this is often misleading and may even prove to be hazardous to health. It is further mentionable that the knowledge on identification and recognition of the various medicinal plants is acquired from those people which may again lead to errors in many cases.

A matter of still greater concern is perhaps to procure the materials at the moment when they are urgently needed. As there is a saying that "Jack found out the telephone number of the fire-station on searching for half an hour after his house was on fire", so also we move out to search bryophyllum or such plants after we sustain cuts and bleed on the body parts. The friend of Ram, Rahim or John may rush here and there to procure the healing plant for him but come back disappointed. They may have procured such a plant but the plant may have been attacked by insect, pest or disease and thus, itself is not a healthy material. It is also likely that in a hurry-scurry, his friend has brought such a plant which was growing alongside a sewerage. As a result, within a few days of application, an inflammation may be eventuated on the injured part as a consequence of infection by the germs carried by the plants as vectors.

From the foregoing discussion, it is apparent that the following aspects should in particular, be given attention to for practical use of plants as medicines by the common people of India.

(*i*) It should be clearly known which plant species are efficacious for which diseases or are capable to protect against which diseases.

(*ii*) Whether any sub-species, variety or type is known within the species which has greater efficacy.

(*iii*) Which specific parts of the plants are to be used for the purpose are needed to be known.

(*iv*) The maturity stage of the plant that is to be used is necessary to be confirmed.

(*v*) How the material should be used, *i.e.*, in fresh or dried form or on extraction with water, oil, ghee, honey etc. must be known to the user.

(*vi*) Whether it is necessary to mix two or more plant species together is a pertinent aspect which the user should take note of.

(*vii*) Whether the plants to be used are available ready at hand, *i.e.*, within a relatively short time should not be disregarded.

(*viii*) Above all, it is essential that the plant themselves are free from the attack by insects or diseases, free from chemical and other pollutants and should be grown in sanitary conditions such that those could be safely used without any adverse side-effect.

In order to fulfil the above conditions, it is necessary that (*i*) the knowledge should be made known to the users, *i.e.*, the common people and (*ii*) the plants are to be grown under controlled condition only, taking care that only the genuine species, varieties etc. of the concerned plants are grown, besides the fact that those are to be grown in hygienic environment and without application of any such material that may act as a source of pollution.

Evidently, this is not always possible if the plant materials used for medicine are procured from other sources. On the other hand, genuine and safe-to-use materials are obtainable if the users grow them under their supervision. For this purpose, it seems necessary that the common people, *i.e.*, the users themselves should maintain plantations of their own where varieties of medicinal plants are to be grown under their direct supervision. Obviously, this will be of great help but it needs pointing out that the land that is available to one may not be enough to grow them. The practicabality is still lesser in urban areas due to scarcity of land and high price of the same.

However, instead of maintaining the plantations of medicinal plants individually by the people, these can be set up and maintained by the municipality, development authority, community, group, institution, organization etc. Thus, in an urban or municipal area, one such plantation may be maintained in each ward by the municipality which would cater to the requirements of the residents in that ward. Similarly, schools, colleges, offices, courts, police-lines, clubs, societies etc. can also maintain such plantations for use by the students or the concerned persons as the case may be, provided open land is available. The surplus products of such gardens may even be sold to the public or pharmaceutical concerns.

In the rural parts of India, establishment of herbal gardens by the panchayats, co-operative societies, schools, cottage-industry centres seeks immense justification particularly as other sorts of medical facility is not adequately available at all places besides that, availability of land to set up the gardens is also not so acute a problem in most parts. A garden maintained by the panchayat may provide materials for the villagers belonged to that, a garden run by a cooperative society may meet the requirements of the members and the like.

Wherever a herbal garden is maintained whether in rural or urban areas, it should be a vital step to pay attention especially on the following three aspects.

(*i*) As many medicinal plants as possible should be grown in the garden. In principle, it should be remembered that a minimum area of about 8 square metre be maintained for each species of plant.

(*ii*) Utmost sanitary measures should be ensured in growing the plants avoiding any contamination of harmful and unhealthy agents as far as possible.

(*iii*) Any chemical fertilizer, pesticide, plant growth regulator or other form of chemical should be avoided to come in contact with the plants and the soil of the garden. Keeping this viewpoint, cultivation procedure of the various medicinal plants presented in this text has been described without application of any such agro-chemical.

Chapter 2

Principles of Establishment

It should be remembered that unlike other types of gardens, a herbal garden should be set up keeping in view a number of specific aspects. The owner of such a garden should pay heed to the following conditions in particular, before such a garden is going to be established.

2.1 Size of the Garden

The garden may be of any size and the area would depend upon certain factors, notably, availability of land, number of persons who would use it, availability of fund and the management capacity. In general, it may be said that a minimum of about 0.06 hectare area becomes necessary to set up such a garden in most cases.

2.2 Selection of Site

A herbal garden may virtually be of little benefit if it is set up in an improper place. Therefore, the following aspects should especially be considered in selecting the site of such a garden.

(1) Nearness to the Users

The garden should be located within easy reach of the users. This is with the idea that the users can reach there easily and at a short time when necessity of procurement of the materials is felt. If it is owned by the panchayat in the village, the location should as far as possible, be close to the panchayat office for in such case, regular watch by the panchayat members would also be done effectively.

(2) Physiography

A flat land should always be given preference in selecting the site. This is because, in an undulated or slopy land, the water and nutrients present in the soil are leached to the depressed parts and accordingly, the elevated areas are deprived. Elevation of the watertable in the depressed parts that may result also hampers drainage of the plants grown there. The land may be selected if the undulations are not much, such that it may be flattened by soil shifting process.

In the hilly terrain however, flat lands are difficult to obtain and in such situations, suitable terraces may be done in order to grow the different types of plants.

(3) Availability of Sunlight

The herbal garden should be located in an open, sunny situation. As majority of the medicinal plants grow best in full sunlight, a land which receives at least 8 hours of sunlight in a day should be preferred. A land where part of it receives partial shade may be considered with the idea that the shade-loving plants may be grown there.

(4) Freedom from Damage by Grazing Animals

The entry of domestic or wild animals into the herbal garden for grazing brings about serious damage to the crops grown there. Hence, an area which is frequently visited by such animals could not be considered to be a desirable site.

(5) Irrigational Facility

It is desirable that the garden should have its own arrangement for irrigation. If this is not possible, irrigation facility near the garden is definitely a desirable feature, provided that the irrigation from that source could be available without difficulty and above all, the irrigation water does not contain toxic substances above the permitted level.

(6) Soil Condition

A very important consideration in selecting the site of a herbal garden is suitability of the soil. While some types of soil are ideally suitable for cultivation of many of the common medicinal plants, some soils are less suitable while some offer to have still lesser suitability. The latter two types of soil may though be brought to a cultivatable condition in some cases, but this is likely to involve much expenditure.

The following conditions however, need to be considered as regards soil condition of the site of a herbal garden.

(a) Elevation

The upland may be considered as ideally suitable for cropping of most of the common medicinal plants. A medium upland may also be considered suitable in some cases but a low-lying or very low-lying land offers little suitability. In such land, the water-table is near the soil surface and becomes still nearer in rainy-season for which drainage of water becomes a serious problem in a low-lying land. Some medicinal plants which are not hampered by poor drainage, *e.g.*, *Cyperus rotundus*, *Eclipta alba* etc. may though be grown in such type of land but plants which develop thick and fleshy roots could in no case, be considered suitable to grow in such a land.

(b) Textural condition

The loam or sandy-loam is no doubt, the best type of soil for growing the medicinal plants except a few where soil of clayee texture may have some suitability. It needs pointing out that soils having higher clay content are unsuitable for growing such plants which develop thick and fleshy roots. The textural condition of the soil may however, be improved to a considerable extent by regular application of organic manure in relatively high amount over some years.

(c) Impermeable stratum

Presence of hard pan in the sub-soil is a great impediment of growing crops. This hampers vertical growth of the roots of the plants and also drainage, eventuating stunted growth of the above-ground parts of the plants. Before choosing the land, it is therefore, necessary to dig a soil-profile and examine the strata of the sub-soil as well.

(d) Soil Reaction

As a large number of medicinal plants grow best in soils of neutral, near neutral or those of partly acidic reactions, such type of soils appear to be congenial. However, it needs pointing out in this connection that soil-reaction of the cropping plots where the plants would be grown is of actual concern rather than the entire land. Besides, the reaction of the soil is also possible to be changed to bring to suitable pH value by judicious application of soil amendments like lime, gypsum, sulphur dust etc. and hence, soil-reaction could not be regarded to be a serious bottleneck unless the soil is persistent with much of lime-nodules, black alkali etc.

(e) Fertility Status

The fertility of the soil is no doubt, an important factor to crop the medicinal plants but again it should be taken note of the fact that the fertility of the actual cropping plots where the plants are to be grown needs consideration rather than the entire land and above all, enriching fertility of the soil is possible to be accomplished by application of plant nutrients in the form of manure and fertilizers. Nevertheless, extremely poor soil could be regarded to have little suitability to set up a herbal garden unless the fertility is at first sufficiently improved in it.

(g) Freedom from Dust

In some places such as near thermal power stations, factories etc., it is seen that dust particles, coal ashes etc. discharged by those are blown away in air and leave residues on the surfaces of the plants. The plants growing along unmetalled roads are also seen to be covered with dust in many places. Such type of deposition of these materials over leaves and other parts of the plants hampers transpiration, photosynthesis and respiration of the plants and thus, seriously hamper their growth. The particles also act as pollutants over the medicinal plants and thereby, hamper their usefulness. Such a site could not therefore, be regarded to be suitable in setting up the garden.

(h) Availability of Labourers

If the garden is of small size, the owners themselves can take part in doing the soil works. This may however, not become possible where the garden is of large size and in such case, labourers are needed to be employed for carrying out the field works. Thus, whether labourers are available should be ensured when a herbal garden covering a large area of land has been planned to be set up.

(i) Freedom from Dispute

The land that is to be used to set up the herbal garden should however, be free from any type of legal disputation such that no objection arises from anybody in its use.

2.3 Selection of Plants to be Grown

The medicinal including aromatic plants are extremely large in number. There is a saying that each and every plant existing in the world has at least some medicinal or nutritive value to man. However, it is not practicable in most cases to introduce a large number of medicinal plants in a herbal garden. Therefore, in the matter of selection of plants, those which are usually of greater necessity should be given preference. Much attention should also be given to grow such plants which are particularly needed for ailments of the children and the elderly people. Besides, for some ailments which break out in particular season, the antidotal plants if any grow in that season should no doubt, be given emphasis for growing.

In a general manner, the owner of the garden should be guided by the principle that is, the number of species of plants that are to be grown should be more while the number of plants belonged to a species may be less.

2.4 Protection against Trespassing

After the land has been possessed or selected to set up the herbal garden, the next immediate step should be to demarcate its area and adopt measures to prevent entry of trespassers and animals. Both can be done together and a cheap and effective method may be to grow hedge plants along its boundaries.

A number of hedge plants are there among which the thorny or spiny ones afford greater protection. Some of the thorny, protective, hardy and easy to grow hedges that may be grown with success are century plant (*Agave americana* and related species), *duranta* (*Duranta plumieri*), Manila tamarind (*Inga dulcis*), henna or *mehendi* (*Lawsonia alba*), *chotra* (*Lantana camara*), *karonda* (*Carissa carandas*), cactus (*Opuntia dillenia*), succulents (*Euphorbia* species), wild rose (*Rosa multiflora* etc.)

There are some hedge plants which have medicinal valve as well, *e.g.*, *Aloe indica*, *Lawsonia alba*, *Calotropis* species, some succulents etc. and these may be considered for growing as hedges to get the extra benefit. A semi-woody climber plant, *viz.*, cowage plant (*Mucuna prurita*) which has great medicinal value if allowed to grow on hedge plants will afford great protection against trespassers as the pods of this plant are provided with hairs which easily sting on the skin of a person whenever touch and results in severe irritation.

Instead of a single row, if two or more rows are set at close spacing between rows and plants afford no doubt, greater protection. However, instead of hedges, fencing with barbed wire, inter-woven wires or even inter-woven barbed wires fitted with angle-iron rods or coal-tar painted bamboo poles may also be erected but these involve higher cost. Where greater protection becomes necessary, a row of thorny hedge on either side of a plain barbed wire or an interwoven barbed wire fencing may be maintained. Digging 30–40 cm wide trench and heaping the dug up soil along the trench is also an effective device to ward off entry of animals. Even rectangular stone slabs may be set in line along the boundaries, if those are locally available at cheap price.

2.5 Preparation of Land

After demarcating the land and making arrangement to prevent entry of trespassing in it, the owner of the garden should start for preparing the land. For this purpose, the following steps should be followed.

(1) Removal of Unwanted Objects

The land possessed for the garden may contain trees, broken buildings or hutments, rubbles, rubbish, papers, plastic materials etc. at the soil surface or at the sub-soil. Evidently, these should be completely removed out from the land before any soil work is done there. If any tree is existent, it should be cut out with root and branch, ensuring that no thick root remains present in the underground.

(2) Flattening

If the soil is not flat, it should be made so by ploughing, spading and levelling with wooden plank or iron-roller. If depressions of greater depth are noticeable, these should be filled by shifting soil.

(3) Control of Animal Pests

The land obtained for the herbal garden may be infested with a number of animal pests that are liable to hamper cropping of the medicinal plants. These are needed to be controlled before layout and plating are done in it. For this purpose, mechanical removal of the agents or use of suitable biopesticide is advisable.

In the following has been presented some of the biopesticides having effectiveness against pests, *e.g.*, mites, termites and nematodes.

(*i*) *Aphid*–Spraying of neem oil or pongamia oil

(*ii*) *Root knot nematode*–Application of neem cake at the time of soil preparation.

(*iii*) *Mites and termites*–Application of neem cake at the time of soil preparation.

(4) Soil Sterlization

The soil may contain many pathogenic micro-organisms also and it is advisable to control them before planting. These pathogens may be of various fungal species, *e.g.*, those of *Fusarium, Pythium, Phytophthora, Rhizoctonia, Armillaria* etc. or bacteria, notably, *Agrobacterium* species. They infect the plants and cause them to wilt, *i.e.*, drying or rottening of the lower part of the stems or dropping of leaves or various other injurious symptoms.

To control these pathogenic micro-organisms, the soil may be heated either directly with electrically heated coils or passing steam from a boiler. Heating should be done for about half an hour, maintaining a temperature of about 60°C both on the surface layer and especially in the sub-soil.

However, heating is a hazardous procedure and hence, chemical method of soil sterilization is largely followed for cultivation of crops. Most of these chemicals that are used emanate volatile fumes which kill the pathogens almost instantaneously. Some of the chemicals that are commonly used include Chloropicrin, Methyl-bromide, Mylone, Formaldehyde, Vapam, etc. While killing the pathogenic micro-organisms, they kill animal pests also. If any snake inhabits in the soil which though is not a pest to any plant is also repelled or killed by the fumes of the above chemicals.

The fumes released by the said chemicals are however, highly toxic to the human beings. Therefore, these should be applied with utmost precaution and the operator should use a mask and spectacles to avoid inhalation of the fume or coming in contact with eyes.

As long as the fumes remain present under the surface soil, they kill the plants if grown there. Therefore, it becomes necessary to wipe out the fumes completely before any planting is done on the land. This should be done by spading the soil or stirring with a hoe few times at interval of several days. Ploughing the land deeply for two or three times at interval of several days is also effective to expel the fumes completely from the land.

Apart from the fumigant chemicals, some other chemicals may also be used for the purpose but the fumigants are much more effective, besides the fact that when they are completely volatilized, no residue is left unlike the non-fumigant chemicals which are effective on direct contact.

2.6 Layout of Garden

Layout of the garden should be done making provision of accessories and the cropping plots in it as stated in the following.

(1) Accessories

The accessories to be maintained in a herbal garden depend in fact, on its area and activities. Nevertheless, the following accessories are considered necessary for even a small garden that measures an area of not more than 0.06 hectare.

(a) Irrigation Arrangement

It is desirable that the garden maintains its own irrigation system. If the area of the garden is small, one or more wells or hand-operated tubewells may be all that is necessary but in a fairly large-sized garden, these may not be enough and a shallow-tubewell would become more effective. For conveying irrigation water to the cropping plots, plastic tubes are better than digging irrigation channels as the latter necessitate some space in the garden. The drip or sprinkler types of irrigation are no doubt, much more efficient than other irrigation systems and make much economy of water, although the initial cost for installation is high.

(b) Nursery

The herbal garden should maintain a nursery of its own. It is not necessary that the nursery should be a large one and its size should be in consistence with the size of the garden and the activities. For a garden of 0.06 hectare, a nursery of 12–13 sq. meter appears to be sufficient. The nursery is meant for raising seedlings, inducing rooting of cuttings and related purposes. A semi-shady situation may be utilized to maintain the nursery.

(c) Office Room

An office room is necessary to be maintained in the herbal garden. Information on the medicinal plants grown in the garden, method of their culture, in which ailments those should be used, mode of their use and other relevant information should be maintained in separate registers in this room. A display board in the office room, stating the plants and their uses will no doubt, be of much help to the users.

(d) Manure-pits

One or more pits become necessary to be maintained in the garden to prepare compost manure. The size of each pit may vary but depth should not be more than 1 meter and it should be provided with thatched roofing. It is better if the pits are made of concrete. The pits should however, be located away from the cropping plots such that the plants grown in the plots are not infected with pests or diseases from the manure source.

(e) Bee-keeping sets

Apiculture in a herbal garden proves to be of great benefit. It does not occupy space but provide honey which has great medicinal value. Besides, the bees also help pollination of flowers of many plant species.

(f) Paths

The necessity of paths and alleys in a herbal garden cannot be disregarded. However, these should be laid out only where these are necessary to be made. The paths should not be unnecessarily wide and should not occupy much space of the garden.

(g) Other Accessories

In addition to the above, other accessories may also be installed by the owner if so felt. Even aesthetic objects like fountains, statutes, rockeries, lily-pools, benches, chairs etc. may be maintained depending on the availability of land and choice of the owner.

(2) Cropping Plots

The cropping plots in the herbal garden are meant for actual cultivation of the medicinal plants in it. These should be located in sunny places and as far as possible along the paths. The size of a cropping plot varies and would depend upon the species of plants, requirements by the users and other factors. It should be noted that in most cases, it is a better practice if the number of plots are made more but size of each plot is not large.

2.7 Procurement of Propagating Materials

The propagating materials should be procured only from a reliable nursery. It should be remembered that it is a wise decision to procure the genuine type of planting materials from a nursery of repute even if the cost is higher than to procure low-graded materials at cheap rate.

The genuiness in respect of the species, variety or type of the materials should in no case be doubtful. The materials should also be healthy and free from attack by insect or animal pests or diseases. In case of seedlings and vegetatively propagated plants, the following aspects should particularly be checked.

(*i*) The material should maintain adequate roots.

(*ii*) Chlorosis or any undesirable symptom is not seen in the material.

(*iii*) It should have good vigour.

(*iv*) The age of the material should be as desired.

Sometimes budded or grafted materials become necessary to be used for planting. In such cases, it should be ensured that graft-union of such a material is sufficiently strong, no callus has developed at the scionic junction and neither the rootstock nor the scion has overgrown that of the scion or the rootstock.

Where seeds are used for raising seedlings for medicinal plants, it should be ensured that they are not dead or damaged, are fully mature, bold and have high viability. It is a better practice to test the viability and vitality of the seeds on conducting germination tests before these are actually sown to raise the seedlings.

2.8 Sowing, Transplanting or Planting

To raise seedlings of some species, it becomes necessary to sow the seeds directly in the plots *in situ* as they cannot withstand transplanting. If the seeds are of bigger size, the common practice is to sow them under the surface at a depth of 1–5 cm depending on the size of the seeds. It is better if such seeds are pre-soaked in water before sowing and sow them maintaining spacing as desired. The seeds which are very small in size are usually broadcast on soil surface and then covered with a layer of soil. After the seedlings emerge, it becomes necessary to thin them out at interval of few days to avoid congestion which results in lanky growth of them as many of such type of seedlings do not survive.

However, transplanting is always better than direct sowing as it produces healthy, sturdy and stout seedlings. To raise seedlings for transplanting, seed-beds are necessary to be prepared which should be raised above the ground and should be located at the nursery of the garden.

The rooted seedlings, cuttings or budded or grafted materials are usually planted directly in the plots maintaining desired spacing.

For most of the medicinal plants except those which grow in tropical region, sowing or planting as the case may be done when growth activity is maximum, *i.e.*, in rainy season or spring. In the rainy season, the plants set well and watering does not become unnecessary unless there is a long period of rainless weather. However, sowing or planting in rainy-season may result in water-logging for which the seeds or the plants may be killed. Therefore, for such materials, which are sensitive to water, stagnation, sowing or planting should be done at the beginning or end of rainy season respectively in low or high rainfall areas. For temperate plants, planting may be done from autumn to winter or spring depending on the species, material used and prevailing temperature.

2.9 Post-planting Care

After sowing of seeds or planting of other propagating materials, adequate care is necessary for survival and vigorous growth of the plants. For such purpose, attention should be given on the following aspects in particular.

(1) Watering

At the early stage of growth for majority of plants, heavy irrigation should be avoided. For such plants, irrigation should be given more frequently but with lesser amount. Sprinkling water through rose-can is satisfactory, if drip or sprinkler irrigation systems could not be installed.

(2) Shading of Plants

Many plants are killed at infant stages due to scorching heat or strong sunshine or both. Therefore, these should be protected with thatches made up of bamboo slices, dried leaves and branches or roofing made with polythene sheet around each plant.

(3) Drainage

In case, water is stagnated around any plant as may happen in rainy season, the water should be drained out without delay.

(4) Weeding

Regular weeding with root and branch after planting should be considered as an essential operation. Hand-weeding is by far, the best method for the purpose.

(5) Mulching

Mulching especially with organic materials is greatly helpful to the young plants in conserving soil moisture, preventing weed growth and also to protect the soil against high or low temperature.

(6) Thinning

For seedling plants, regular thinning becomes necessary to avoid congestion, which as stated earlier makes the seedlings tall in appearance.

(7) Plant Protection Measures

Regular checking of each and every plant becomes necessary after planting and any insect or disease affected part should be clipped with secateurs as soon as detectable. Application of a biopesticide made with a decoction of tobacco leaves, *neem* leaves, turmeric powder, chilli powder, black cumin seeds, *vitex* leaves, vasaka leaves, bay leaves, asafoetida etc. in suitable proportions at desired intervals gives effective control of aphids and other minor pests. It is not advisable to apply chemical pesticides on the plants of a harbal garden as far as possible.

(8) Replacement in Mortality

Some plants may die at the early stage of their growth. The garden owner should regularly visit each and every cropping plot to check the plants grown there and whenever there is any mortality, it should be replaced by another.

Chapter 3
Principles of Management

As the plants that are grown in a herbal garden are exclusively used as medicines, some special precautions become necessary to be maintained in respect of their cultivation and management.

Among others, the following measures are of particular significance which should be kept in view in maintaining such a plantation.

3.1 Sanitary Condition

It is essential that a hygienic condition should be maintained in every part of the garden. Thus, whenever any extraneous material is necessary to be introduced into the garden, care should be taken that it should not be a source of microbial or chemical pollution. It should be noted that the implements that are to be used in the garden should only be used for plants grown in the garden itself and should not be taken outside for other purposes. It is also advisable that after working with, the implements should be washed, dipped in potassium permanganate solution and put in place.

Any organic material such as leaves or twigs, manure and even feathers of birds fallen here and there in the garden may be a source of infection and hence, these should be removed as soon as come to sight.

It is even desirable if separate shoes or other footwears are maintained for persons exclusively for the purpose of working or roaming about in the garden. The persons desirous to take samples should also enter with these footwears.

The owner(s) and users of the garden should in fact, be very particular that a sanitary environment prevails in all parts and corners of the herbal garden.

3.2 Nutrition of Plants

As far as possible, use of chemical fertilizers should be avoided in a herbal garden. Although in some parts of the text, use of chemical fertilizers has been stated, those may be replaced by equivalent proportions of organic manure. However, even if chemical fertilizers become necessary to be applied, mild doses may be used, avoiding any promiscuous application of the same.

Among organic manure, green-manuring by raising leguminous plants in the cropping plots and burying those in the soil at early stage of their growth is beyond doubt, a good practice to enrich fertility of the soil and also to improve its textural condition. This should be done once a year and if not possible, at interval of one or more years. Use of bacterial fertilizer is also of much help to restore fertility of the soil.

3.3 Intercultural Operations

To encourage growth of the plants, regular intercultural works become necessary to be done in the cropping plots. The weeds take up large amount of moisture and nutrients from the soil for which the plants in cultivation are to suffer competition and the latter make poor growth. Therefore, regular weeding is an essential operation that is to be done in each cropping plot. It should be taken note of the fact that the operation should be done manually by uprooting the weeds and any chemical weedicide should never be applied for purpose in a herbal garden.

Sometimes it is noticeable that along with weeds, some rogue plants also make their way in the cropping plots. These plants usually belong to the allied species or genera of the cultivated plants and sometimes it may even be difficult to distinguish these plants from those of the cultivated plants that are grown in the plots. Very careful observations are therefore, necessary and whenever such an off-type plant is visualized, it should be rooted out and removed from the garden.

Along with weeding, regular hoeing of the soil in the cropping plots proves to be of great benefit. This should be done by stirring the soil lightly with a hand-hoe or any suitable device. By improving aeration of the soil, hoeing improves greatly to boost up growth of the plants.

Mulching, *i.e.*, covering the soil with other materials is no doubt, an effective method to conserve moisture content of the soil and disallow the growth of weeds. It is advisable to do the operation preferably with an organic material and more than one material may be run together and mulched. Use of wood-ash along with the mulching materials is also a good practice which adds potassium to the soil.

3.4 Irrigations

Irrigation in a cropping plot should be done with careful judgement, ensuring that it is neither under-irrigated nor over-irrigated. This can be accomplished by observing the moisture status of the soil and the condition of the plants. The following three aspects should particularly be given attention to in this regard.

(*i*) The irrigation water should not contain any chemical that is either toxic to the plants or to the human beings. If necessary, the water may even be filtered and used.

(*ii*) To irrigate medicinal plants, sprinkling irrigation is no doubt, most desirable. By doing so, the leaves and other parts of the plants are washed for which the dust and dirt collected over them are removed out. As a result, the rate of transpiration, respiration and photosynthesis are increased eventuating higher metabolic activity and growth of the plants. The insect eggs, larvae, pupae etc. if attack the plants are also washed away by sprinkling water.

More importantly, as the leaves or other plant parts are made free from insect eggs, larvae, pupae or dust particles, they are rendered to a much safer condition for medicinal use.

(*iii*) While irrigating a plot, care should be taken that water does not stagnate in it for more than ten minutes. If such happens, the stagnated water needs to be drained out without delay. The same practice should be done when there is heavy downpour in the rainy season, which may result in water-logging in the plot.

3.5 Training and Pruning of Plants

Training refers to imparting a particular size, shape or form to a plant while pruning of it refers to function, *i.e.*, primarily aims at flowering of it. While in pruning operation, it is essential that the parts of the plant like stem, branches, twigs, leaves, flowers etc. are to be cut off, in training, it may or may not become necessary. Since shape, size or form is obviously changed to a greater or lesser extent whenever pruning is done to a plant, training is automatically done to it by pruning. But without cutting of any part, a plant is possible to be trained.

The medicinal plants that are grown in the herbal garden may be of various species and various forms. That is, some may be trees, some shrubs, some herbs, creepers, ramblers etc. and accordingly, their growth habit are not same. In accordance with, training of these plants should be done to suit the conditions.

For those plants, which are creeping in habit, extra support becomes necessary for their creeping. To make so, scaffolding may be done to enable them to creep over those. The scaffolding may be done with poles and slices of bamboo tied together firmly with rope but permanent structures of such type may also be built up with iron rods and galvanized wires and these are of permanent nature unlike the former ones. Some creeping plants and especially those of rambler types, may even be crept on trees or shrubs.

In case of some plants, it is noticeable that they grow more in lengthwise manner, *i.e.*, assume taller appearance without producing much side-shoots. Physiologically, the condition is referred to as apical dominance, denoting that the apex of the plant dominates suppressing the growth of branches. In case of such type of growth of the plants, the apical part of the plant which consists of the terminal bud is to be removed by clipping and this effectuates growth and spread of the branches below it.

To encourage more side branches, the apical buds at the end of the branches should also be clipped and this would ensure increased branching from the shoots.

If over-crowding of plants is noticed such that adequate light and air fail to enter in the inside of the plants, it may become necessary to thin out some plants by uprooting those, maintaining desirable spacing. This may also be done by encouraging upward growth of the plants by allowing to grow the terminal buds undisturbed and disallowing much side growths by shortening the length of the branches.

For some plants from which flowers or fruits are required, it is sometimes noticed that the upper part of the branches bear these while the lower parts remain barren. This is particularly seen in many upright growing shoots of shrubs that produce flowers in their axils. By artificially bending those upward growing shoots to grow horizontally or form like arches by suitably tying with strong rope, flowers may be induced at their lower parts also.

There are again some plants, shrubs or trees which produce flowers at the newly born or younger aged shoots unlike others which bear on mature shoots. In both the cases, flower-bearing shoots become necessary to be encouraged to enhance flowering when flowers or fruits become necessary for use as herbal drugs. To accomplish this, plant parts are needed to be pruned adjusting the time judiciously such that sufficient number of shoots become available for flowering. Similarly, to secure flowers or fruits over a prolonged period, it may become necessary to prune out a little quantity of the flowers or fruits as the case may be at early stage of their growth.

It should be noted that whenever a plant part is cut off, it leads to entry of pathogenic microbes through the cut surface until a crust is formed over it which requires some days. Therefore, after cutting of any plant part, the cut surface should immediately be covered with a disinfecting material to prevent entry of pathogens in the manner as stated below under the heading, 3.7 (Taking Samples).

3.6 Post-planting Measures

The various medicinal plants that are grown in a herbal garden are meant for use as therapeutic or prophylactic agents by the human beings against diseases, disorders and wounds. With this objective, the plants in such a garden should be grown with great care ensuring that they do not contain any extraneous chemical substance which may cause harm to the users. This is of particular significance as many of the plants may have to be used by the children who are more vulnerable to the chemical pollutants that are associated with them. Many of these plants may become necessary to be applied in eyes or genitals also which are even more susceptible organs against toxins. Therefore, to get rid of such chemical contamination, it is desirable that the plants should be grown without application of any chemical, meaning thereby that an organic system of farming be adopted.

With this concept, the requirement of nutrients by the plants should be met up by copious application of non-toxic organic agro-input, dispensing with inorganic organs. Even in the selection of organic manure also, such materials which may add undesirable chemical should be refrained from application.

Toxicity is however, much greater by the use of the chemical forms of pesticides. In accordance with, it is warrantable that no chemical pesticides be added to the crops to control pests and diseases. In fact, an integrated pest management needs to be implemented in a herbal garden. This should no doubt, be an environmentally healthy approach employing the available skills, cultural practices, mechanical and biological control.

Some of the methods that may be adopted to control pests and diseases in these plants without deposition of toxic chemicals have been stated in the following.

(a) Hand-picking

Removal of plant parts stuck with eggs, larvae, pupae etc. of insects or those showing disease symptoms by hand is beyond doubt, the safest and highly effective method. For this purpose, a can containing little of kerosene should be taken and the affected parts on explanting should be placed in it and covered with lid. On making such collection, the container should be emptied by throwing out the materials outside the garden and may even be burned.

The process appears to be slow but can be done at lesser time and effectively if carried out regularly at an interval of few days.

(a) Washing with Water

Irrigation by sprinkling wash away may insect eggs, larvae etc. adhering on leaves and other plant parts. The method is more effective if the water is discharged with high pressure through a blower and delivered both on upper and lower surfaces of leaves. Where the garden is of small size, washing the leaves and the plants with hand may also be done.

(b) Broom-trap

Hanging brooms here and there in the garden is an effective means as many insects especially those of nocturnal habit take shelter in the brooms. At day time, each broom wherein insects have taken shelter be placed in a suitable bag and vigorously shaken so as to collect the insects in that.

(c) Inverted Umbrella

Holding an umbrella in an inverted manner below a shrub or a tree and shaking the branches is a good means to collect aphids and some other insects or their larvae or pupae inside the umbrella.

(d) Light-trap

Placing burning lamps carefully at suitable distances from the plants is known to cause burning of light-loving insects.

(e) Scare-crow

Birds may be scared by erecting scare-crows in the garden.

(f) Banding with Cloth

Wrapping the lower parts of the stem of the plants with polythene or cloth near ground level is a highly effective methods to control the pest, known as mealy-bug. The insect which dwells in the soil cannot cross the banding by crawling and thereby, the plants are saved from its attack.

(g) Sprinkling Wood-ash

Occasional sprinkling of wood-ash on the cropping plots is a highly effective means to control many insects pests and diseases. But it should be noted that the ash to be used should not be of coal as this may kill the plants. Wood-ash is no doubt, safest but it should not be applied in rudimentary stage of growth of the plants and in no case, this should be applied in high amount as it may cause death of the plants.

(h) Application of Neem-cake

The oil-cake made from seeds of *neem* (*Azadirachta indica*) is a highly effective device to control many soil-borne insects, termites, nematodes and pathogenic fungi. On application, this should be thoroughly incorporated into the soil with the help of a hoe.

(*i*) Application of Home-made Pesticides

As stated earlier, suitable pesticide can be prepared by boiling leaves of *neem*, tobacco, bay, custard apple, fern, jatropha, notchi, vasaka, vitex, ipomea etc., paste of ginger and garlic, roots of *Cyperus rotundus*, powders of turmeric, chilli, black cumin and asafoetida in suitable proportions. On cooling, this should be strained, mixed with little of non-alkaline soap (*e.g.*, soap-nut) as sticking agent and sprayed or sprinkled over the plant. Although not all, but many of the minor insect pests and diseases may be controlled by this.

(j) Biological Control

Some insects are known to be predators in that they themselves are not pests to the crops grown but feed on other insects which act as pests. Some examples are *Chrysoperia carnea, Malada astur, Podisus maculiventris, Cantheoconidia furcellata* etc., which predate on many insects. Maintenance of them where possible is a good measure to control the pests. Many birds like crows, herons, fowls etc. also feed on insect larvae and pupae. Rearing poultry birds and pigeons is advised by many to control insect pests of crop plants.

(k) Prophylactic Measure

Above all, it is a known fact that prevention is better than cure and hence, adoption of sanitary measure as stated earlier cannot be disregarded to prevent attack by many insect pests and diseases.

3.7 Taking Samples

Not only in cultivation and management of the garden but much care should be taken while taking samples from the plants for the purpose of medicinal use.

Attention should particularly be taken on the following aspects when samples are to be taken from the plants.

(*i*) Only that part of the plant which is necessary should be explanted without disturbing other parts.

(*ii*) The amount of material that is actually required should be taken without making wastage of much amount.

(*iii*) Explanting of the plant parts should be done with a

convenient secateur, pliers or scissiors and that should be disinfected by dipping in potassium permanganate solution before use.

(*iv*) Plant parts should be taken by giving flat cuts avoiding bruising.

(*v*) After cutting of twigs or branches, the cut surfaces should be smeared with a paste made from lime and turmeric powder to avoid pathogenic infection to the plant through the cut surfaces. (Fungicidal pastes are however, available for the purpose but those are not advisable for medicinal plants because of containing copper).

Chapter 4

Cultivation of Plants and their Medicinal Properties

As stated earlier, almost every plant in the world has some medicinal properties. The prophylactic and curative properties against ailments of human beings have though been known for many plants, a large number remains to be explored.

In the following has been presented the general cultivation procedure of only a few medicinal plants, which appear to have greater appositeness to include in a small–or medium-sized herbal garden in different parts of India.

4.1 *Bhumyamalaki*

Botanical Name

Phyllanthus niruri Linn.

Indian Names

Sanskrit–Bhumyamalaki, Bahupatri; *Hindi*–Jaramla, Jangli Amli, Bhuinanvalah, Bhonyabali; *Bengali*–Bhui Amla, Sadahazur-mani; *Marathi*–Bhuivali; *Gujarati*–Bhonya Anmali; *Telugu*–Nela Usirika; *Tamil*–Keela Nelli; *Kannada*–Nela Nelli, Kiranelli Gida; *Malayali*–Kizha Nelli; *Orissi*–Bhui Anola, Badianla.

Botanical Family

Euphorbiaceae.

Suitable Places for Growing in India

The plants grow abundantly throughout India upto 700 m altitude during rainy season, however, with less frequency in Southern part of the country. It can be successfully grown in Utttar Pradesh, Haryana, Punjab, Maharashtra, Tamil Nadu, Kerala, Andhra Pradesh, Karnataka, Bihar, Orissa, West Bengal etc.

Botanical Description

Plant

Annual herb of 30–60 cm high, quite glabrous.

Stem

Stem often branched at the base, angular, leaf-bearing branchelets slender, spreading.

Leaves

Leaves numerous, subsessile, distichous often imbricating, 6–13 by 3–6 mm, elliptic-oblong, obtuse (rarely subacute), glaucous beneath, base rounded; petioles very short; stipules lanceolate-subulate, very acute.

Flowers

Flowers small, monoecious, very numerous, axilary; yellowish green.

Male Flowers

1–3 in branch, fascicled, subsessile.

Calyx

Sepals-4, free, imbricate, 0.6 mm long, rounded.

Corolla

Absent.

Androecium

Stamens 3; in the centre of the flower; filaments free; anthers 2-celled, sessile on a short column, parallel, dehiscence extrorse. Disk present with minute glands.

Female Flowers

Female flower solitary.

Calyx

Sepals-4, free, imbricate, 1.2 mm long, oblong, subacute with white margins, not enlarged in fruit.

Corolla

Absent.

Gynoecium

Ovary usually 3-celled; ovules 2 in each cell; styles minute, free, usually 2 fid, with slender arms. Disk annular, lobed.

Fruit

Capsules 2.5 mm diam., depressed-globose, smooth, scarcely lobed.

Seeds

Seeds 1.5 mm long, trigonous, rounded and with longitudinal regular parallel ribs on the back.

Species and Varieties

At present there is no named or certified varieties under this crop under cultivation.

Plant Parts Used

Whole plant.

Chemical Component

The dried leaves contain 0.4 per cent of a toxic bitter principle, phyllanthin, traces of a tasteless substance, hypophyllanthin and about 5 per cent of a colourless wax made up mostly of esters (85 per cent) of long chain fatty acids and alcohols, free fatty acids and hydrocarbons. Phyllanthin is toxic to fish and frog. The leaves are rich in potassium (83 per cent, fresh basis) which is considered responsible for their powerful diuretic effect.

Stem contains saponin. A decoction of the stem and leaves dyes cotton black; sometimes it is substituted for ink. Alcoholic extracts of leaves and roots show antibacterial activity against *Micrococcus pyogenes* Var. *aureus* and *Escherichia coli*.

Cultivation Procedure

Soil

Phyllanthus niruri is found to be well-adapted to a wide variety of soils and at alkaline to acidic pH. Much damage of the plant is not found under water-logged condition.

Climatic Requirement

The plant is a tropical weed and rarely survives under very low temperature conditions.

Method of Propagation

The plants are generally propagated by seeds. Fresh, healthy seeds are sown in the nursery and about 1 kg of seeds are enough for production of seedlings to transplant an hectare area of land. For raising seedings, the seeds are sown in well-prepared nursery beds. Well-decomposed farmyard manure (FYM) should be mixed with top layer of the soil while preparing the nursery beds.

Since the seeds are very small, they are usually mixed with dry soil, sand or wood ash to allow uniform distribution of seeds on the nursery bed. Appropriate moisture is necessary to be maintained in the seed-beds till the seeds have germinated. In north Indian plains, the seeds are sown in nursery-beds in the month of April–May.

Seeds germinate within 10–15 days of sowing. Approximately 15–30 days old seedlings, which are about 10 cm tall are ready for transplanting in the field.

Land Preparation

The land is repeatedly ploughed and brought to a fine tilth and weeds, stubbles and pebbles are to be removed. The field is divided into plots of convenient size and the soil is mixed with recommended dose of manures. About 20–25 tones of FYM is required for an hectare area of land. Groundnut cake, bone-meal, rapeseed cake and vermicompost are also beneficial for better growth of the plants. To remove mites and nematods from the field, prior application of neem cake is recommended at the doses of 7–12 kg/ha.

Planting

Transplantation in the field is done maintaining a spacing 15 cm × 15 cm between plants. A plant population of 80,000 plant/

ha is optimum in most cases. A proper irrigation just after transplanting ensures establishment of seedings.

Manuring

In low fertile soil, 20–25 tonns of FYM/ha is recommended but in moderately fertile condition, the dose may be reduced at 15–18 tonns/ha. If irrigation facilities are available, it is recommended to green manure the field with leguminous crops. The seeds of the green manure crop may be treated with the bacterial inoculants before sowing so as to increase the development of root nodules which absorb atmospheric nitrogen and fix it in to the soil.

Irrigation

The plants are drought resistant and do not require much water but irrigations in summer is helpful.

Intercultural Measures

The field should be absolutely free from weeds for which regular hand-weeding at monthly interval is required.

Intercropping

The plants may be grown as an intercrop with any shrub or tree.

Crop Protection Measures

The plants are practically free from the attack of any serious pest or disease.

Harvesting

Plants are harvested when the rainy-season is over and when they are still green and herbaceous. Since the active constituents of the plant accumulate more in the leaves, production of higher leaf-mass is desired for the extraction. Plants harvested in September usually contain highest amount of leaves.

Post-harvest Processing

The harvested plants are cut into pieces in suitable size and dried in shade and suitably stored.

Yield

The total yield of dried herbage goes to 0.5–0.9 tonnes/ha under irrigated condition.

Medicinal Properties

The fruit and the plant are known to be useful in thirst, bronchitis, leprosy, anaemia, urinary disorders, anuria, biliousness, asthma, hiccough, gastric disorders, sores, dysentery, ringworm etc. Besides efficacy in dropsy, gonorrhoea and inflammations of the gastro-intestinal tract is also on record.

An infusion of the young shoots is administered in dysentery. The powdered leaves and roots are pulverised and made into poultice with rice water to lessen oedematous swelling and ulcers.

The fresh root is said to be an excellent remedy for jaundice. In the Konkan region, the root rubbed down with rice water is given as a remedy for menorrhagia.

4.2 Black Nightshade (Syn. Common Nightshade, Garden Nightshade, Hound's Berry, Morelle, Petty Morel)

Botanical Name

Solanum nigram **Linn.**

Indian Names

Sanskrit–Kakmachi; *Hindi*–Makoi; *Bengali*–Gurkamai, Kakmachi, Tulidun; *Gujarati*–Piludi; *Telugu*–Kachchipundu, Kachi, Kamanchi, Gajju Chettu; *Tamil*–Munatakali.

Botanical Family

Solanaceae.

Suitable Places for Growing in India

This plant can be grown throughout India in dry parts, up to an elevation of 2,100 m.

Botanical Description

Plant

A variable annual.

Stem

Stem erect, glabrous or more or less pubescent, much divaricately branched.

Leaves

Leaves numerous, 2.5–9 by 2.5 cm; ovate-lanceolate, subacute or acuminate, glabrous, thin, entire, sinuate toothed, tapering into the petiole; petioles 2 cm long.

Flowers

Flowers small, in extra-axillary subumbellate 3–8 flowered cymes, peduncles 6–20 mm long, slender; pedicels 6–10 mm long, very slender.

Calyx

Calyx 3 mm long, glabrous or nearly so; lobes 5, oblong, obtuse, 1.25 mm long, not enlarged in fruit.

Corolla

Corolla 4–8 mm long, divided more than ½ way down into 5 oblong subacute lobes.

Androecium

Filaments short, flattened, hairy at the base; anthers 2.5 mm long, yellow, oblong, obtuse, notched at the apex.

Gynoecium

Ovary globose, glabrous; style cylindric, hairy.

Fruit

Berry 6 mm diam.; globose, usually purplish black, but sometimes red or yellow, smooth, shinning.

Seeds

Discoid seeds, 1.5 mm diam., minutedy pitted, yellow.

Species and Varieties

At present there is no named or certified varieties under this crop under cultivation.

Plant Parts Used

Whole plant and fruit.

Chemical Component

Analysis of leaves gave the following values: moisture (82.1 per cent), protein (5.9 per cent), fat (1.0 per cent), total minerals (2.1 per cent), carbohydrate (8.9 per cent), calcium–410 mg/100 g, phosphorus–70 mg/100g, iron–20.5 mg/100 g. Leaf is a rich source of riboflavin; the values for various vitamins present in the leaf are–riboflavin–0.59 mg/100 g, nicotinic acid–0.92 mg/100 g, vitamin C–11.0 mg/100 g. Leaves contain β-carotene 0.74 mg/100 g & α-carotene content is negligible. Citric acid is present in 5 per cent.

Fruit contains glucose and fructose (15–20 per cent), vitamin C and β-carotene. Green unripe fruits, however, contain glycoalkaloids and their eating is a toxic hazard to human beings as well as livestock. Ripe fruit contains very little alkaloids and can be consumed without ill-effects. Seeds contain 17.5 per cent protein in dry weight basis. Seed produces a greenish yellow oil (21.5 per cent) The fatty acid component of the oil are–linoleic (46.63 per cent); oleic (49.73 per cent); palmitic (1.76 per cent) and stearic (1.88 per cent) The unsaponifiable matter contains sitosterol.

Immature green fruit of the plant contains four steroidal glycoalkaloids, *viz.* solamargine, solasonine and α–and β–solanigrine; all of them yield solasdine as the aglycone. It also contains a steroidal genin, tigogenin. Solamargine and solasonine ae present also in leaves. The total alkaloid content of fruits and leaves are 0.101 per cent and 0.431 per cent respectively.

Cultivation Procedure

Soil

The plant is very hardy and thrives in different kinds of soil including dry, stony, shallow or deep ones. It grows as a weed throughout dry parts of India. Deep sandy loam to loamy soils of medium fertility is however, preferred for its large-scale cultivation.

Climatic Requirements

The distribution of the plant makes it apparent that there is no specificity in its climatic requirements. It comes up well in tropical and subtropical areas. However, the growth in tropical areas is better than in the subtropical areas, where its growth is slow due to low temperature in winter. The crop prefers warm, dry conditions all round the year and remains for 150–180 days in field. Where rainfall is high and well-distributed, it can be grown as a rainfed crop. It can be successfully grown up to an elevation of 1,300 m above sea-level.

Method of Propagation

Propagation is mostly done from seeds.

Fresh seeds collected from healthy ripe fruits are sown in well-prepared, raised nursery beds in April–May by broadcasting in rows at 8–10 cm apart and at about 1.5 cm depth. They are then covered with a light soil and leaf-mould mixture at 1: 1 ratio and watered to keep the bed moist. For one hectare area of land, 500 g of seeds are sufficient. The seeds germinate within 15–20 days after sowing.

The 25–30 days-old seedlings which are 12–15 cm tall are ready for transplanting.

Land Preparation

The land is repeatedly ploughed and brought to a fine tilth and weeds, stubbles and pebbles are to be removed. The field is divided into plots of convenient size and the soil is mixed with recommended dose of manures. About 20–25 tones of FYM is required for an hectare area of land. Groundnut cake, bone-meal, rapeseed cake and vermicompost are also beneficial for better growth of the plant. To remove mites and nematods from the field, prior application of neem cake is recommended at the doses of 7–12 kg/ha.

Planting

The seedlings are transplanted in rows at 60 cm apart in well-prepared field. A plant population of 40,000 plants/ha is optimum.

Manuring

In low fertile soil, 20–25 tonns of FYM/ha is recommended but in moderately fertile condition, the dose may be reduced at 15–18 tonns/ha. If irrigation facilities are available, it is recommended to green manure the field with leguminous crops. The seeds of the green manure crop may be treated with the bacterial inoculants before sowing so as to increase the development of root nodules which absorb atmospheric nitrogen and fix it into the soil.

Irrigation

The plants are drought resistant and do not require much water but irrigation in summer is helpful.

Intercultural Measures

The crop responds well by 2–3 periodic hoeing and weeding at interval of 20 or 30 days. Mulching with rice straw or cut-grass is recommended to minimise weed growth.

At early flowering stage, the top 2 cm portions of the plant are removed to promote vegetative growth and enhance the alkaloid content.

Intercropping

The plants may be grown as an intercrop with any shrub or tree.

Crop Protection Measures

The plants are practically free from the attack of any serious pest or disease.

Harvesting

The crop is ready for harvest after 150–180 days of transplanting. The plants are cut about 3–4 cm above the ground level and dried in shade.

Post-harvest Processing

The harvested plants are cut into pieces and dried in shade and stored in gunny bags.

Yield

The total yield goes to 0.8–1.2 tonnes/ha under rainfed condition and may increase to 1.5–1.7 tonnes for an irrigated crop.

Medicinal Properties

The berries are known to be oleaginous, pungent, laxative, alterative, aphrodisiac, diuretic and improve appetite. They are useful in diseases of the heart and the eye, in pains, piles, inflammation, "tridosh", leucoderma, itch, worms in the ear, dysentery, hiccough, vomiting, asthma, bronchitis, fever, urinary discharges etc.

The root bark is laxative and used in diseases of the ear, eye and the nose. It is efficacious in ulcers on the neck, burning of the throat, inflammation of the liver, chronic fever, gripes but not to be given to pregnant women.

The leaves which have bad odour and taste are used for headache and diseases of the nose.

The fruit is effective in thirst due to fever and inflammatory condition.

The seeds are laxative and useful in giddiness, gonorrhoea, thirst and different types of inflammations.

In West Bengal, the berries are used in fever, diarrhoea, eye diseases, rabies etc.

In Maharastra, six to eight ounce of juice of berries is given for treatment of chronic enlargement of liver and is considered a valuable alterative.

In north-western provinces, the juice is used in blood-spitting, piles, dysentery while in the Konkan, the young shoots are given in chronic skin diseases and psoriasis..

The juice of the leaves is used by the Chinese people to alleviate pain in inflammation of the kidneys and bladder and also in gonorrhoea.

4.3 Blond Psyllium (Syn. Isapaghula, Spogel Seeds)

Botanical Name

***Plantago ovata* Forsk.**

Indian Names

Hindi–Isubgol; *Bengali*–Eshopgol; *Marathi*–Isabgola; *Gujarati*–Isapghol, Ghoda Jeeru, Umto Jeeru; *Telugu*–Isapgola Virtulu; *Tamil*–Iskolvirai; *Kannada*–Isafgolu, Visamagolu; *Malayali*–Karkatasringi.

Botanical Family

Plantaginaceae.

Suitable Places for Growing in India

It is commercially cultivated in the districts of Banaskantha and Mehsana in North Gujarat. It is also grown to a very small extent in Patiala and Hissar districts of Punjab and in Uttar Pradesh.

Botanical Description

Plant

A stemless or nearly stemless, softly hairy or woody scapigerous annual.

Leaves

Leaves 7.5–23 cm long, scarcely reaching 6 mm broad, narrowly linear or filiform, finely acuminate, entire or distantly toothed, attenuated at the base, usually 3-nurved.

Flowers

Scapes axilary, longer or shorter than the leaves, glabrous or pubescent. Flowers in ovoid or cylindric spikes of 1.3–3.8 cm long; bracts 4 mm long and about as broad as long, broadly ovate or suborbicular, concave, membranous, except the narrow midrib, glabrous; flowers small, greenish, dimorphic.

Calyx

Sepal 4, imbricate in bud, persistent; calyx 3 mm long usually glabrous; sepals elliptic, obtuse, concave, scarious except the midrib which is as broad (or nearly so) in the inner as in the outer sepals.

Corolla

Corolla scarious, hypogynous; lobes 4, short, imbrecate in bud, corolla-lobes rounded, 3 mm long, concave, obtuse, apiculate, glabrous.

Androecium

Stamens 4, inserted on the coralla tube; filaments filiform, persistent; anthers large, pendulous, versatile, 2-celled.

Gynoecium

Ovary superior, 2-celled, ovules one in each cell, axile placentation; style simple.

Fruit

Capsul 8 mm long, ellipsoid, obtuse, the upper half comming off as a blunt conical lid, membranous, glabrous, 1–4-celled, circumscissilely dehiscent.

Seeds

Seed usually attached by the centre; testa thin, mercilaginous; albumen fleshy; embryo cylendric, transverse; radical inferior. Seed 3 mm long, avoid oblong, boat-shaped, smooth and yellowish.

Species and Varieties

Gujarat Isabgol 2 (GI 2), GI -1, Niharika, Jawahar Isabgol 4 (JI 4), Haryana Isabgol 5 (HI 5) are some high yielding varities which are recommended for large scale commercial cultivation.

Plant Parts Used

Seeds.

Chemical Component

The mucilage of *isabgol* is colloidal in nature and its composition varies with the condition of preparation. It is mainly composed of xylose, arabinose and galacturonic acid, rhamnose and galactose have also been reported. Two polysaccharide fractions have been separated from the mucilage. One fraction (uronic acid 20 per cent) is soluble in cold water and on hydrolysis yields d-xylose (46 per cent), an aldobiouronic acid (40 per cent), *l*-arabinose (7 per cent), and insoluble residue (2 per cent); the other fraction uronic acid (3 per cent) is soluble in hot water forming a highly viscous in solution which sets to a gel on cooling and yields on hydrolysis *d*-xylose. (80 per cent), *l*-arabinose (14 per cent), aldobiouronic acid (0.3 per cent), and trace of *d*-galactose.

The seeds contain in addition to mucilage, a semidrying fatty oil (0.5 per cent), small amounts of aucubin, and tannin, and an active principle exhibiting acetylcholine-like action. The fatty oil solidifies at –8°C, and has a bright yellow colour. The constituent fatty acids in the oil are: linolenic (0.2 per cent), linoleic (47.9 per cent), Oleic (36.7 per cent), palmitic (3.7 per cent), steric (6.9 per cent) and lignoceric (0.8 per cent) acid. The embryo yields 14.7 per cent of a linoleic acid-rich oil, linoleic acid (53.4 per cent) whose use has been suggested as a dietary hypocholesterolemic agent in place of corn oil. Feeding of the embryo oil as dietary supplement for lowering the serum cholesterol level gave encouraging results in experimental animals.

Cultivation Procedure

Soil

The crop is usually grown in light sandy or sandy-loam soils but also thrives well in clay loam, medium black, black cotton and heavy black soils. Good drainage is an essential feature for its successful cultivation in heavy soils. The crop is also able to withstand a low level of soil salanity. In general, a silty-loam soil, having a soil pH from 4.7 to 7.7 with low nitrogen and moisture content, is considered more suitable for rich growth of the plants and high yield of the seeds.

Climatic Requirements

Isabgol grows very well in cool and dry climate. It is cultivated as an irrigated crop in winter season which remains in the field for about 4 months.

Sowing seeds during the first week of November is found to give higher yield. Sowing early in the season especially with a higher seed rate makes the crop vulnerable to downy mildew diseases. Late sowing usually provides a shorter period of growth in winter along with the possibility of seed-shattering which is due to the summer rains occuriring in April–May. If the weather is humid at maturity, the seeds shatter, resulting in low yield. Heavy dew or even a light shower decrease the yield considerably and sometimes may even lead to a total loss of the crop. The temperature required for maximum seed germination is around 25°C.

Method of Propagation

Isabgol is conventionally cultivated by sowing seeds. Seeds which are bold, healthy and from previous year's crop should be used for sowing. A seed rate of 4 kg per hectare is usually sufficient for good plant stand. Higher seeds rate is not desirable as it encourages downy mildew disease.

Direct sowing by broadcasting is practiced but line sowing with a spacing of 30 cm × 5 cm helps in better intercultural operations.

The seeds may be mixed with fine sand or sieved FYM while sowing. After sowing, the field is covered by light sweeping with a broom or tree twig having foliage and the sweeping should be done in one direction only. To facilitate germination, care should be taken in placement of seeds in the soil so that they do not get buried deep into the soil.

The sowing should immediately be followed by light irrigation or sprinkling. Germination starts 4–5 days after sowing but if delayed, it should be stimulated by another watering.

For sowing seeds, last week of October to second week of November is considered as ideal.

Land Preparation

After harvest of the kharif crop, the land is brought to free of weeds, clods and have fine tilth. The number of ploughings, harrowings and hoeings that are to be done depend upon the soil conditions, the previous crop and the extent of weed infestations. FYM amounting to 10–15 tonnes/ha should be incorporated into the soil at last ploughing. The field should be divided into suitable plots of convenient size in accordance with the texture of the soil, slope of the field and the source and amount of irrigation water. For light soils in flat land, a plot size of 8.0 m × 3.0 m is considered most suitable.

Planting

Isapaghula are generally transplanted in the field after 20–30 days of germination at 30 cm × 30 cm spacing where transplanting method are being followed. But commercially direct sowing method of cultivation is recommended.

Manuring

Soil application of well-rotten FYM at the rate of 5–10 tonnes/ha appear to be sufficient to secure optimum yield of the crop.

Irrigation

A light irrigation should be given immediately after sowing. With heavy irrigation the seeds are carried to one end of the field and get buried deep into the soil. This results in poor growth of the plants. If germination is poor 6–7 days after sowing, a second irrigation is advisable. In general, three irrigations are required for the crop which are at sowing, followed by one each at 30 and 70 days after sowing. The last irrigation should be given when the maximum number of spikes are in milking stage. Irrigations should be scheduled when soil moisture level goes 20–25 per cent below the field capacity.

Intercultural Measures

The first weeding should be done after 20–25 days of sowing. Ordinarily 2–3 weedings within two months of sowing are sufficient to keep the weeds under control.

Intercropping

Other crops may be grown along with isabgol which do not provide shade on the main crop.

Crop Protection Measures

The following pest and disease infestations are found in the Isabgol field:

(1) *Downy Mildew*

Early sowing, higher seed rate, frequent irrigation make the crop more susceptible to this disease, caused by the fungal species, *Peronospora plantaginis* and *P. alta*. Normally the disease appears at the time of spike-initiation. The first symptom appears as small patches on the leaves, which spread and completely destroy those. The disease spreads rapidly in humid weather. It is very difficult to keep the disease under control once it has affected the crop severely.

(2) *Damping-off Disease*

The causal organisms are *Pythium ultimum, Rhizoctonia solani* and *Fusarium oxysporum* which appear at the seedling stage of the plants.

(3) *Powdery Mildew*

This disease appears at flowering time due to attack by the fungus, *Erysiphe cichoracearum*.

(4) *Aphid Attack*

Apis gossypii generally appears 60–70 days after sowing.

(5) *White Grubs Attack*

White grubs are reported to damage the roots of young plants.

(6) *Termites Attack*

Termites damage the crop by cutting off the root.

Harvesting

The crop takes about 110–120 days to come to maturity. At maturity, *i.e.* in March–April, the leaves turn yellowish and spikes brownish in colour. The crop is harvested when plants are fully dried and seeds turn dark brown. The atmosphere should be dry at the time of harvest. It should preferably be done after the dew dries out at about 10 am. To prevent loss of seeds by shattering, slightly unripe spikes can also be harvested if there is possibility of unseasonal rain but the husk quality deteriorates from such harvest.

Harvesting is done by cutting the plants at the ground level or by uprooting those when the soil is very loose.

Post-harvest Processing

The harvested plants are brought to the threshing floor, bundled in large cloth pieces and spread out. After a few days, seeds are threshed by trampling using tractor or bullockes. The seeds are also threshed by tractor operated threshing machine. Threshing should be done during the early morning so as to facilitate easy separation of the seeds from the spikes. Sometimes, water is sprinkled over the heap to facilitate easy threshing. Care should be taken not to apply excess water as it spoils the quality of the produce. The straw of the crop is used as a cattle-feed. The plants are threshed and winnowing is done till they become clean. (The seeds may be marketed as such or the husks sold separately)

To remove the husks from the seeds, the seeds are passed 6–7 times through stone-grinders, sieved and screened through several graded mesh.

Most of the exported type of husk is of the grade which is designated as 70 mesh. The highest quality husk is white with no particles of red kernels. The husks obtained (total yield 26–27 per cent) from different millings vary in quality. They are kept separately and mixed in different proportions according to the quality of demand.

Yield

Gujarat Isabgol-1 variety yields 800–900 kg of seeds/ha, while the new variety, Gujarat Isabgol-2 yields 1000 kg of seeds/ha.

Medicinal Properties

The seeds are sweetish, acrid, highly mucilaginous, astringent to the bowels, tonic and are useful in biliousness, dysentery and leprosy. They are also useful in inflammatory and bilious derangements of the digestive organs and applied as poultice to rheumatic and gouty swellings. The decoction is useful in cough and chronic diarrrhoea. When moistened with water, they form a good emollient poultice.

The seeds yield to water a good deal of mucilage and this form a cooling demulcent drink which is prescribed in cases where emollients are required. A slight degree of astrigency and some tonic property may be imparted to the seeds by application of a moderate degree of heat.

The poultice made from the crushed seeds with vinegar and oil are applied to rheumatic and gouty swellings. Two or three drachms of seed suitably moistened with warm water and mixed with sugar if necessary are given in dysentery and irritation of the intestinal canal to exert easy bowel movement. The roasted seeds have an astringent effect and are useful in irritation of the bowels and dysentery.

The seeds are highly beneficial in chronic dysenteries of amoebic and bacillary origin and chronic diarrhoea due to irritative conditions of the gastro-intestinal tract. A glucoside named aucubin has been found in the seeds, but it is not physiologically active. The action of the drug appears to be purely mechanical, being due to the large amount of mucilage which is present in the superficial layers of the seeds. The mucilage is not acted on by the digestive enzymes, and therefore, passes through the small intestine in unchanged state. It lines the mucous membrane of this part of the gut and its demulcent properties give it a protective and sedative effect. Practically the whole of the mucilage is passed out unchanged during the 12 to 24 hours following its administration. When it passes through the gut, it coats the inflammed and ulcerated mucosa and protects it from being irritated by the fluids and gases which are the products of gastro-intestinal and bacterial digestion. The toxins that are present in the gut are further absorbed by the gel and their absorption into the system is prevented. The seeds are taken up in large quantity and as they swell up in contact with water, they increase the bulk of the intestinal contents. Thereby, it relieves chronic constipation by mechanically stimulating the intestinal peristalsis. The mucilage of the seeds in believed to act in very much the same way as liquid paraffin but is free from any injurious effect.

4.4 Comphire (Syn. Cypress Shrub, Egyptian Privet, Henna Plant, Jamaica Mignonette, Mindie, Tree Mignonette)

Botanical Name

Lawsonia inermis Linn.

Indian Names

Sanskrit–Mendika, Raktgarbha, Ragangi; Arb. –Henna, Al Khanna; *Hindi*–Mehndi; *Bengali*–Mehedi, Mendi; *Marathi*–Mendhi; *Gujarati*–Medi, Mendi; *Telugu*–Goranti; *Tamil*–Marithondi, Maruthani; *Kannada*–Mayilanchi, Gorante; *Malayali*–Mailanchi, Pontlasi; *Orissi*–Benjati.

Botanical Family

Lythraceae.

Suitable Places for Growing in India

It can be cultivated in tropical and warm temperate region. It is cultivated commercially mainly in Punjab, Gujarat, Madhya Pradesh and Rajasthan. The major important centres of production are Faridabad in Gurgaon district (Punjab), Bardoli and Madhi in Surat district (Gujarat), Pali, Sojat and Nagor district (Rajasthan)

Botanical Description

Plant

A glabrous much-branched shrub.

Stem

Stem softly woody; lateral branches 4-gonous, often ending in a spinous point.

Leaves

Leaves 1.3–3.2 by 0.6–1.6 cm, entire, opposite, elliptic or broadly lanceolate, acute or obtuse, often mucronulate, base tapering; petioles very short or absent.

Flowers

Flowers numerous, less than 1.3 cm across, fragrant, white or rose-coloured, in large, terminal pyramidal panicled cymes; pedicels short, slender.

Calyx

Calyx 3–5 mm long, broadly campanulate, lobes 4, 2.5–3.1 mm long, broadly ovate, acute.

Corolla

Petals 4, very shortly clawed, inserted at the top of the calyx tube; 3 mm long, as broad as long, suborbicular or subreniform, undulate.

Androecium

Stamens 8, inserted in pairs on the calyx tube opposite the calyx-lobes; anthers broadly oblong, the connective thick.

Gynoecium

Ovary superior, subglobose, 2-4 celled; ovules many, axile placentation; style thick, stightly longer than stamens; stigma capitate.

Fruit

Capsule 6–6.5 mm diam., globose, slightly veined outside, supported by the persistent calyx and tipped with the style, coriaceous, irregularly breaking up, ultimately one celled.

Seeds

Seeds closely packed on a central placenta, angular, trigono-pyramidal, about 2.5 mm long, externally subtuberculate.

Species and Varieties

Two varieties are known, *viz.* Hinna (odorous) and Rajni (more colouring)

Plant Parts Used

Leaves.

Chemical Component

The leaves contain tannin, lawsone, glucose, gallic acid, fat, resin, mucilage, alkaloid etc. The flowers have strong aroma and yield essential oil on steam-distillation. The seeds are rich in fatty acids, carbohydrates, proteins, wax and other material.

Analysis of air-dried leaf powder gave the following average values: moisture (8.97 per cent); ash (14.85 per cent); and tannin (10.21 per cent) The tannin content appears to be very variable; a sample from Jammu & Kashmir contained 4.9 per cent tannin. Henna contains 25–33 per cent water-soluble matter; aqueous solutions are orange in colour and show a green fluorescence. The principal colouring matter is lawsone, 2-hydroxy-1: 4-naphthaquinone which is present in dried leaves in a concentration of 1.0–1.4 per cent. Henna extracts are useful for dyeing in acid baths; alkalis intensify the colour but destroy the dyeing properties.

Besides lawsone, other constituents present in henna are: gallic acid, glucose, mannitol, fat, resin (2 per cent), mucilage and traces of an alkaloid.

The flowers of henna plant have a strong aroma and yield on steam-distillation, 0.01–0.02 per cent of an essential oil with brown or dark brown colour and a strong fragrance suggestive of tea rose. Henna or *mehendi* oil has been used in perfumery since ancient times. It consists mainly (90 per cent) of α–and β-ionones (ratio 1: 4); a nitrogenous compound and a resin are present. Extraction of flowers with benzene yields 1.65 per cent of a simi-solid concrete with an agreeable odour, somewhat phenolic and very tenacious.

Analysis of henna seeds gave the following values: moisture (10.6 per cent); protein (5.0 per cent); fatty oil (10–11 per cent); carbohydrates (33.62 per cent); fibre (33.55 per cent) and ash (4.75 per cent) Extraction of the seeds with petroleum ether yields a non drying viscous oil. The fatty acid composition of the oil is as follows: behenic (1.69 per cent); arachidic (9.6 per cent); stearic (15.78 per cent); palmitic (9.07 per cent); oleic (34.66 per cent) and linoleic (29.31 per cent) The unsaponified matter contains waxes and colouring matter. The oil is reported to be used in Uganda for anointing the body. The root contains a red colouring matter.

Cultivation Procedure

Soil

The henna plants may be grown in almost any type of soil, from light loam to clay loam, but it does best in heavy soil which is retentive of moisture. It can also tolerate a little alkalinity in the soil.

Climatic Requirements

The plant requires a hot, moist climate and an elevation between 100 and 1000 m. It can be easily grown even in areas which receives heavy rainfall with high relative humidity.

Method of Propagation

Propagation may be done from seeds and stem cuttings, but the former method is recommended for commercial purpose.

Propagation by Seed

The seeds have hard covering and hence, they are at first soaked in water for 20–25 days with frequent changes of water to facilitate sprouting (the average germination is 20 per cent) The sprouted seeds are usually mixed with fine sand and broadcast in well-prepared nursery beds during March–April. The seedbeds are kept moist and kept free from weeds. The seedlings grow to 20–30 cm height in the next 3 months and then they are transplanted in wet fields during the monsoon season (in July–August)

Propagation by Cuttings

Terminal stem cuttings obtained from one year old growth with 3–5 internodes show better rooting than those which are from older shoots. Rooting of the cuttings may be done in polythene bags filled with the common pot mixture.

The cuttings may be planted in April–May and by that, they will be ready for planting in field by August.

Land Preparation

The land should be ploughed and brought to a fine tilth and leveled at least one month before. Weeds, stubbles and pebbles are to be removed. For convenience, the field is divided into plots of convenient size and the soil is mixed with recommended doses of manures. The land should be applied with 40 tonnes of FYM.

Planting

The plantlets may be set singly or 2–3 together in holes at a spacing of 15 × 30 cm or 30 × 30 cm.

Manuring

About 2 tonnes of FYM in 2 split doses is recommended annually to boost up vegetative growth of the plants for commercial cultivation.

Irrigation

Daily irrigation is necessary at the early stage of growth. After successful establishment, the field should be irrigated fortnightly. Sprinkler system of irrigation may be adopted for economising the irrigation water.

Intercultural Measures

During the first year of planting, weeding and hoeing are done when weed growth is found in the field. After the application of FYM to the pits, earthing-up is done from the channels. Pruning may be done before rainy season for better vegetative growth.

Intercropping

Henna is mainly cultivated as a hedge plant. However, it can also been grown as an intercrop with rose, jasminum and other ornamental or medicinal plants.

Crop Protection Measures

Hena plants may be affected by the following pests

(1) *Termite Attack*

Young and mature plants are affected by this insects. They damage the crop by cutting off the root.

(2) *Mites Attack*

Velvetty layer may be visible on the leaves.

Harvesting

The plants in their third year of growth begin to yield the leaves and continue to produce economic yields for the next 25 years or so. Normally, 2 harvests are taken, *viz.* in March–April and in October–November. Leafy branches are cut near the ground level and dried preferably in shade.

Post-harvest Processing

The dry branches are beaten on the ground for collecting the leaf crop.

Yield

The average yield of henna under rain-fed condition is about 1 tonne per hectare. Higher yield upto 2.5 tonnes per hectare is obtained when the raised as an irrigated crop. The harvest during October–November (summer crop) accounts for 75–85 per cent of the total annual yield.

Medicinal Properties

The leaves of henna are emetic, expectorant, allay burning sensation and helpful in leucoderma. They are considered as diuretic, and useful in headache, hemicrania, lumbago, bronchitis, boils, ulcers, stomatitis, ophthalmia, syphilitic sores, amenorrhoea, scabies, diseases of the spleen, enrich the blood, favour the growth of the hair. The flowers are vulnerary, an infusion cures headache. The seeds act as tonic to the brain.

The bark of the plant is given in jaundice and enlargement of the spleen, in calculous affections and as an alterative in leprosy and obstinate skin diseases. The decoction is applied in burns, scalds etc.

The decoction made from the leaves is used as an astringent gargle in relaxed sore throat. The fresh leaves are also rubbed over the soles of the feet in the diseases known as burning of the feet. A paste of it is made with vinegar which is used for the same purpose. Henna is used as an emollient poultice and the flowers are considered refrigerant. The flowers are also used as a soporific, being for this purpose placed in a pillow. The oil and essence are rubbed over the body to keep the body cool.

4.5 Country Borage (Syn. Indian Borage)

Botanical Name

Coleus amboinicus **Lour.**, *C. aromaticus* **Berth.**

Indian Names

Sanskrit–Pashanabhedi; *Hindi*–Pathorchur; *Bengali*–Patherchur; *Marathi*–Pathurchur; *Tamil*–Karpuravalli; *Kannada*–Makandiberu.

Botanical Family

Labiatae.

Suitable Places for Growing in India

It is well grown in subtropical Himalayan regions from Kumayun to Nepal, Bihar and the Deccan plateau of Southern India. It is commercially cultivated in parts of Rajasthan, Maharastra, Karnataka and Tamil Nadu.

Botanical Description

Plant

A perennial herb wity tuberous rootstock, shrubby below, hispidly villous or tomentose.

Stem

30–90 cm long, quardrangular, fleshy.

Leaves

Leaves 2.5–5 cm, petioled, broadly ovate or cordate, crenate, fleshy, very aromatic, exstipulate.

Flowers

Flowers in lax or close paniculate or racemose, densely 6–10 flowered cymes, shortly pedicelled, 3 mm long, whorls distant.

Calyx

Sepals 5, connate in a 2-lipped calyx, upper lip widest, not decurrent, ovate, acute, membranous, lower lip acuminate, calyx throat villious within, enlarged in fruit.

Corolla

Petals 5, connate in a 2-lipped corolla, pale purplish, tube short, exserted, decurved; throat inflated, equal or obliquely swollen; upper lip short, broad, 4-fid, recurved; lower lip much longer, entire, boat-shaped, stipitate or narrowed at the base.

Androecium

Stamens 4, didynamous, declinate, shortly exserted, connate below into a sheath separate from the corolla; filaments simple, anther-cells usually fonfluent. Disk enlarged in front.

Gynoecium

Ovary superior, deeply 4-partite; style simple from the centre of the ovary between the lobes, erect; stigma 2-fid; ovules solitary in each lobe of the ovary, erect, anatropous.

Fruit

Fruit of 4-orbicular or ovoid smooth dry nutlets; basal scar small; fruiting calyx suberect.

Seed

Seed solitary in the nutlets, small, erect, albumen scanty, embryo conform to the seed; radicle inferior.

Species and Varieties

Coleus barbatus Benth. and *C. tuberosus* Benth. are also grown in different parts of India. K-8 is a high yielding variety recommended for commercial cultivation. "Selection–K" a nonflowering type has been found good under Karnataka conditions.

Plant Parts Used

Tubers.

Chemical Component

The tuberous roots of the plant are found to be rich source of forskolin or coleonol.

Cultivation Procedure

Soil

It thrives better in porous and well drained soils with a ph ranging from 5.5 to 7. However, it does not require very fertile soils and can be economically grown even on the soils with marginal fertility. The red sandy soils of Karnataka are ideal for the cultivation of this crop.

Climatic Requirements

Coleus is a crop of tropics and found growing well at an altitude of about 2400 m under tropical and subtropical conditions. It prefers humid climate with RH ranging from 83 to 95 percent and a temperature range between 10–25°C for its successful growth. The annual rainfal in such areas ranges from 100 to 160 cm, mainly during June to September months. It is also found to perform well in less humid and warmer regions when grown as an irrigated crop.

Method of Propagation

Coleus can be propagated by seeds as well as by stem cuttings. For commercial plantings the crop is propagated through terminal cuttings. For this purpose about 10–12 cm long cuttings comprising 3–4 pairs of leaves are preferred. Such cuttings and planted in well prepared nursery beds under shade and regular care about watering is taken. As there is no problem in rooting they establish well in nursery. After about a month's time when the cutting were produced sufficient roots they are ready for transplanting.

Land Preparation

The land is repeatedly ploughed and brought to a fine tilth and weeds, stubbles and pebbles are to be removed. The field is divided into plots of convenient size and the soil is mixed with recommended dose of manures. About 20–25 tones of FYM is required for an hectare area of land. Groundnut cake, bone meal, rapeseed cake and vermicompost are also beneficial for better growth of the plants. To remove the mites and nematods from the field, prior application of neem cake is recommendate at the doses of 7–12 kg/ha.

Planting

The spacing between the plants are recommended as 60 cm × 20 cm apart from each plant.

Manuring

In low fertile soil, 20–25 tonns of FYM/ha is recommended but in moderately fertile soil, the dose may be reduced at 15–18 tonns/ha. If irrigation facilities are available, it is recommended to green manure the field with leguminous crops. The seeds of the green manure crop may be treated with the bacterial inoculants prior to sowing to increase the development of root nodules which absorb atmospheric nitrogen and fix it in the soil.

Irrigation

The first irrigation is given immediately after transplanting, if there are no rains. During the first two weeks after planting, the crop is irrigated once in three days and, thereafter, weekly irrigation is enough to obtain good growth and yield.

Intercultural Measures

Due to frequent irrigation during the initial stages there is a lot of competition from weeds. In order to obtain economic yield frequent weeding during the early growth period is desirable. Further, as the plants cover the soil under their foliage, not much are of weeding is required.

Crop Protection Measures

Coleus crop is sufficiently hardy and relatively free from the damages due to pests and diseases. However, in some areas, the crop faces some attack, which are as follows.

(1) *Leaf Eating Caterpillar Attack*

Pyralid caterpillar (*Glyphodes vertumnalis*) causes appreciable damage to the leaves. The caterpillars roll leaf and feed on the green matter. Some other caterpillars (*Daphnis nerii* L. and *Dceilophola nerii* L.) are also reported to feed on tender leaves, causing defoliation of the plant.

(2) *Mealy Bug Attack*

During May–June, *Helopeltis theiveora* attacks the vegetative parts and spikes.

(3) *Root Knot Nematodes*

Root knots appear as galls of various sizes, covering the root system. Stunted growth of plants, etiolation and decreases in leaf size are the symptom in the arial portion. The galls, on examination, show the presence of mites, various soil fungi and nematodes (*Heterodera* sp) Generally, brown clay soils supporting the natural growth of the plant are found to be infested with nematodes, while dark clay soils are free from them.

(4) *Bacterial Wilt*

Plants die-back and start drying from the tips. Leaves fall prematurely.

Harvesting

The crop is ready for harvest after about 135–150 days of planting. During the growing period if any flowers are produced they should be nipped off to obtain more biomass. The crop is harvested manually by uprooting the individual plants.

Post-harvest Procesing

The tubers are separated, cleaned and cut into suitable pieces and shade dried for the extraction of "forskolin".

Yield

On an average, an yield of 1500 kg of dried tubers per hectare may be obtained. However, if proper cultivation practices are applied an yield of 2500 kg of dried tubers can be easily obtained per hectare.

Medicinal Properties

The leaves are said to have a specific action on the bladder and to be useful in urinary diseases, vaginal discharges etc. The juice mixed with sugar is given in cases of colic in children, and acts as a powerful aromatic carminative.

Inspite of its intoxicating properties the people of West Bengal employ it in colic and dyspepsia.

In Sri Lanka, a decoction of the leaves is given for asthma, chronic coughs etc.

In China, the juice of the leaves is considered carminative and is given to the children suffering from wind colic. The decoction is given for asthma, chronic bronchitis, epilepsy and convulsions.

4.6 Country-Mallow

Botanical Name

Sida cordifolia **Linn.**

Indian Names

Hindi–Kungyi; *Bengali*–Swetberela, Berela, Bala; *Gujarati*–Bala Baldana, Mahabala, Khapat; *Telugu*–Tellaantisa, Tellagorra, Chirwbenda, Suvarnamu; *Tamil*–Nilatutti, Paniar-tuthi; *Kannada*–Hettuthi, Hettugigada, Kisangi, Chittuharalu; *Malayali*–Kurunthotti, Vellurum, Kathuram; *Orissi*–Badianaula, Bisvokopari; Punjabi–Kowar, Simak.

Botanical Family

Malvaceae.

Suitable Places for Growing in India

The plant is naturally grown in moist places throughout tropical and sub-tropical India, ascending to an altitude of 1,050 m.

Botanical Description

Plant

Shrubby, softly hairy and with much stellate hair nearly all over and subpersistent, downy, erect, 1.5 m high.

Stem

Stem stout with long branches, sometimes rooting at the nodes, bark light yellowish brown.

Leaves

Leaves 2.5–5 cm long, cordate, ovate-oblong, crenate, obtuse or subacute, not acuminate; petioles 1.2–3.8 cm long.

Flowers

Regular, bisexual, pedicels solitary or few together, short, some up to 1.2–2 cm long, jointed much above the middle, solitary, towny-yellow or white.

Calyx

Sepals 5, valvate, connate below of 1/3–1/2 their length, 6–8 mm long, lobes ovate, acute.

Corolla

Corolla small, yellow; petals connate at the base and with staminal tube; corolla slightly exceeding the calyx.

Androecium

Stamens many, monadelphous, filaments numerous, form staminal tube which is divided at the top into numerous antheriferous filament; anthers kidney shaped, dehiscent transversly.

Gynoecium

Ovary 5-celled, strongly reticulated, ciliate on the upper margins, the two dorsal margins almost scabrid; ovule 1 in each cell, pendulous; styles as many as the carpels, stigma terminal.

Fruit

Fruit globose, depressed, enclosed by the calyx; 6–8 mm diam.; carpels 7–10, separating from each other from the central axis, strongly reticulated, ciliated on the upper margins, the two dorsal margins almost scabrid; awns 2 on each carpel, nearly as long as the carpels, linear, retroversely scabrid hairy.

Seeds

Seeds black-chestnut, smooth.

Species and Varieties

At present there is no named or certified varieties under this crop under cultivation.

Plant Parts Used

Root, leaves, seeds.

Chemical Component

The plants contain alkaloids which are maximum in seeds. Ephedrine is a notable alkaloid of the seeds. The seeds also contain a fatty oil (3.23 per cent), steroids, phytosterol, resin, resin acids, mucin and potassium nitrate.

Cultivation Procedure

Soil

A well-drained, sandy-loam to clay-loam soil which is moderately rich in humus is considered suitable for cultivation of this crop.

Climatic Requirements

The plant thrives well in tropical and subtropical climates but the growth in tropical situation is better. It prefers warm and moist condition all round the year and where rainfall is high and well distributed, it can be grown as a rainfed crop. The plants may be successfully grown upto an elevation of 1,050 m.

Method of Propagation

Sida can be grown from seeds or stem cuttings. The plants propagated from cuttings flower earlier than the plants from seed propagated, and hence, it is recommended that for drug production, the plants should preferably be propagated from cuttings.

For seed propagation, one year old seeds should be used as the seeds undergo dormancy. The seeds can either be directly sown in the field *in situ* or in nursery beds and the seedlings emerged out are transplanted in the field. In direct sowing method, the seeds are broadcasted at the rate of 1–1.2 kg/ha at the onset of monsoon in May–June, in lines 80–100 cm apart. After sowing, the land is lightly covered with fine leaf-mould. As the seeds are very small, they are mixed with sand and leaf-mould mixture in 1:1 ratio, about 10 times of their weight and sown. A light irrigation should be given if it does not rain in next 2 days of sowing. Germination takes place after 10–20 days and after 30–45 days of germination, the seedlings are thinned out maintaining a spacing of 80–85 cm within the rows.

For transplanting of seedlings, the one year old seeds are sown in well-prepared, raised nursery beds in March–April by broadcasting in rows spaced 8–10 cm apart and at about 1.5 cm depth. They are then covered with light soil and leaf-mould mixture at 1:1 ratio and watered to keep the bed moist. For nursery sowing 400 g of seeds produces enough seedlings to plant one hectare area of land. The seeds germinate within 10–12 days after sowing and the 60 days-old seedlings which are 15–20 cm tall are ready for transplanting.

In case of vegetative propagation, the stem–cuttings obtained from lateral stems are generally used. Lateral stems which are of one year old and of pencil like thickness give better rooting. Pre-soaking the cuttings overnight in 25–50 ppm NAA solution facilitates rooting.

Land Preparation

The land is repeatedly ploughed and brought to a fine tilth. Weeds, stubbles and pebbles are to be removed. The field is divided into plots of convenient size and the soil is mixed with recommended dose of manures. About 20–25 tones of FYM is required for an hectare area of land. Groundnut cake, bone-meal, rapeseed cake and vermicompost are also beneficial for better growth of the plants. To remove mites and nematods from the field, prior application of neem cake is recommended at the doses of 7–12 kg/ha.

Planting

It is advisable to transplant the seedlings at a spacing of 75 cm × 85 cm apart in the field. A plant population of 20,000 plants/ha is considered adequate in most conditions.

Manuring

In low fertile soil, 20–25 tonns of FYM/ha is recommended but in moderately fertile soil, the dose may be reduced at 15–18 tonns/ha. If irrigation facilities are available, it is recommended to green manure the field with leguminous crops. The seeds of the green manure crop may be treated with the bacterial inoculants before so as increase the development of root nodules which absorb atmospheric nitrogen and fix it into the soil.

Irrigation

The plants are drought-resistant and do not require much water. Also, a majority of the growers raise a rain-fed crop during the monsoon season. Light irrigations are required in case of inadequate rains. The irrigated crop requires 5–6 light irrigations.

Intercultural Measures

The crop is given 2-3 periodic weeding and hoeing at interval of 20 or 30 days. Once the plants covers the field, they smother weed growth. Mulching with rice straw or cut-grass is recommended to minimize if weed growth is large.

At early flowering stage, the top 2 cm portions of the plant are removed to promote vegetative growth and alkaloid content.

Intercropping

The plants may be grown as an intercrop with any tree plantation.

Crop Protection Measures

The plants are practically free from the attack of any serious pest or diseases.

Harvesting

The crop is ready for harvest after about one year of planting. The crop is harvested manually by uprooting the individual plants during the month of May–August.

Post-harvest Processing

Root

The roots are washed properly, then cut into pieces of 15–25 cm length and dried.

Stem

The basal stems upto 10 cm long are separated from roots and cut into pieces and dried.

Leaves

The harvested leaves are dried in shade and stored.

Seeds

Seeds are collected by a light threshing to the dried seed pods of harvested dried plants.

Yield

On an average, an yield of 150 kg of dried roots per hectare may be obtained. However, if proper cultivation practices are applied an yield of 200 kg of dried tubers can be easily obtained per hectare.

Medicinal Properties

The plant is astringent, emollient, aphrodisiac and is effective in cough as a pectoral and belic. The bark is known to cure urinary troubles and discharges. The fruit is acrid and sweet, digestive, cooling, astringent, aphrodisiac and is useful in blood diseases, bleeding piles, diseases of the throat, phthisis and insanity.

A decoction of the root with ginger is given in intermittent fever. It is also administered in fever accompanied by shivering fits and strong heat of body. The powder of the root-bark is given along with milk and sugar for the relief of frequent micturition and leucorrhoea. In diseases of the nervous system, the root is used in combination with other medicines.

The bark of the root mixed with sesamum oil and milk is very efficacious in curing cases of facial paralysis and sciatica when caused by the inflammation of the nerves concerned.

The seeds are used as aphrodisiac, and are administered in gonorrhoea and are also given for colic and tenesmus.

4.7 Creat

Botanical Name

Andrographis paniculata **Nees in Wall.**

Indian Names

Bengali–Kalmegh; *Gujarati*–Kariyatu; *Hindi*–Kalmegh, Karayat, Mahatita; *Kannada*–Nelaberu; *Malayali*–Kiriyattu, Nelaveppu; *Marathi*–Olikiryata; *Orissi*–Bhuinimba; *Sanskrit*–Bhunimba, Kirata; *Tamil*–Nilavembu; *Telugu*–Neelaveemu.

Botanical Family

Acanthaceae.

Suitable Places for Growing in India

It is chiefly found in the plains throughout India from Himachal Pradesh to Assam and Mizoram and all over south India.

Botanical Description

Plant

An erect branched annual, 0.3–0.9 m high.

Stem

Stem erect, branches sharply quadrandgular, often narrowly winged in the upper part, slightly enlarged at the nodes.

Leaves

Leaves 5–7.5 cm by 1.2–2.5 cm, lanceolate, acute, glabrous, slightly undulate, pale beneath; base tapering; main nerves 4–6 pairs, slender; petioles 0–6 mm long.

Flower

Flowers small, solitary, distant, in lax spreading axillary and terminal racemes or panicles, the whole forming a large pyramidal paniculate inflorescence; bracts 2.5–3.0 mm long, lanceolate; bracteoles similar or absent; pedicels 0.8–4.1 mm long, glandular–pubescent.

Calyx

Calyx 3–3.5 mm long; sepals equal, linerar–lanceolate, glandular, pubescent.

Corolla

Corolla rose-coloured, 1–1.2 cm long, hairy outside, 2-lipped rather more than half way down; tube 5–6 mm long, slightly enlarged below the limb; upper lip 4–5 mm long, oblong, 2-toothed at the apex; lower lip equal in length, deeply 3-lobed, the lobes 2.3–2.5 mm long, linear-oblong, subobtuse.

Androecium

Stamens 2; filaments flattened, hairy in the upper part; anthers 2-celled, excerted, the cells oblong, parallel, subequal, muticous, beard at the base.

Gynoecium

Ovary 2 celled; ovules 3–6 in each cell; ovary glabrous; style slightly pubescent, slender; stigma shortly 2-lobed.

Fruit

Capsules 20 mm. by 3 mm, linear–oblong, acute at both ends, compressed contrary to the septum.

Seed

Seeds numerous, hard, subquadrate, osseous rugosely pitted, glabrous, yellowish brown; retinacula lanceolate.

Species and Varieties

At present there is no named or certified varieties under this crop under cultivation.

Plant Parts Used

Whole plant.

Chemical Component

Analysis of whole plant gave the following lactones (dry basis): andrographolide, 0.6 per cent; 14-deoxy-11-oxo-andrographolide, 0.12 per cent; 14-deoxy-11, 12-didehydroandrographolide, 0.06 per cent; 14-deoxyandrographolide, 0.02 per cent; and a non-bitter constituent, neoandrographolide 0.005 per cent. The leaves contain andrographolide (1 per cent) From the petroleum ether extract of the leaves the following alkaloids have been isolated: α-β-unsaturated lactone, homo-andrographolide, andrographosterol, andrographane, andrographone a wax, and two esters containing hydroxyl groups.

The roots gave apigenin-7, 4′-do-O-methyl ether, andrographolide and a new natural flavone. 5-hydroxy-7, 8, 2′, 3′-tetramethoxyllavone. They also contain a monohydroxy-trimethylflavone, andrographin and a dihydroxy-di-methoxyflavone panicolin. The presence of α-sitosterol is also reported.

Cultivation Procedure

Soil

The plant grows abundantly in moist, shady and inferior land and sometimes in dry forests also. It can be grown in almost all types of soil. In native state, it is found to grow in clayey to sandy soils in various locations. However, sandy loam soil which is rich in organic matter is considered better for its growth and yield. The cultivation is difficult in water-logged conditions.

Climatic Requirements

The crop is well-suited to tropical and sub-tropical regions. But cooler climate with well-distributed rainfall are considered ideal.

Studies done at Bangalore have shown that the best season for planting of the crop is during the month of June when it attains maximum growth and this gives highest yield.

With the onset of monsoon, the plant grows luxuriantly and starts flowering during September. In the north Indian plains, flowering and fruiting continue upto December until temperature drops.

Method of Propagation

Creat is propagated either by seed, cutting or layering. But for commercial purpose, the crop is propagated from seed as it is not only easy but economical, compared to the vegetatively grown plants.

Seeds are small and remain dormant for five to six months. They are either sown directly in the main field or in the nursery and then the seedlings are transplanted. About 400 g of seeds are considered enough to plant in a hectare area of land. Seeds are sown in two methods. In the first method, those are sown in polythene bags filled with a mixture of soil, sand and organic manure in 1: 1: 1 proportion. In the other method, the seeds are allowed to germinate directly in nursery beds of $3 \times 1.5 \times 0.15$ m size. The nursery beds are mixed with well-rotten cattle manure @ 20 kg/m^2 for raising healthy seedlings. The beds should be pulverized and levelled during the month of May. The seeds are sown in lines 5 cm apart in the nursery beds. It is advisible to cover the seeds with very thin layer of soil and compost mixture.

Beds should be covered properly by suitable mulch and sprinkled with water regularly. The seedlings emerge within 6–7 days. Immediately after germination, mulch is removed as it causes elongation of the seedlings. After 10–15 days, regular irrigation should be given till the seedlings are ready for planting. Seedlings will be ready for transplanting into the main field when they are 45–50 days old.

Land Preparation

The land is prepared by repeated ploughing and levelling to bring to a fine tilth. About 25 tonnes of FYM per hectare is mixed well with the soil at the time of the last ploughing. The land is laid out into plots of convenient sizes with provision of irrigation channels for easy management.

Planting

For direct sowing, furrows are made at a distance of 30 cm and about 3–4 seeds are sown at one place maintaining a distance of 15 cm between two plants. In the case of seedling transplantation, a spacing of 30 × 15 or 15 × 15 cm is maintained. However, is order to get the maximum herb yield, a spacing of 15 × 15 cm is best.

Transplantation of seedlings is done during the last week of June. Beds should be irrigated immediately after planting.

Manuring

Creat can be grown on poor to moderate fertile soil. But it responds very well to the application of FYM @ 25 tonnes per hectare of land.

Irrigation

The crop is usually grown as rainfed. But in case of long dry periods irrigation at suitable intervals becomes necessary. Irrigation during autumn does not have much benefit on biomass yield as by that time the plants are in reproductive phase.

Intercultural Measures

Creat is a small herbaceous shrub and, therefore, the competition with weeds during its initial stages of growth becomes necessary to be avoided by keeping the land free from weeds.

The first weeding followed by hoeing is done after about 20–30 days of planting. After this, one or two weeding is necessary after 60 days of sowing to keep the weeds under control during the initial stages of crop growth.

Intercropping

The plants may be grown as an intercrop with any shrub or tree.

Crop Protection Measures

Creat is a hardy plant and generally is not attacked by any pest and diseases of a serious nature.

Harvesting

The crop is ready for the first harvest after about 90–120 days of sowing when plants start flowering. Maximum herb biomass can be obtained in 90–100 days after which leaves start shedding. If the plant is raised as annual crop and planted during the month of May–June, it should be harvested by the end of September when flowering starts. At the time of flowering initiation, the active principle, *andrographolide* comes to high level in leaves.

The harvesting is done by cutting the plants at the bases, leaving about 10 –15 cm of the stem for regeneration of new shoots. Top-dressing with biofertilizer may be done to enrich the soil. The regenerated plants are ready for harvest again within about 60 days of the previous harvest. In all, 2–3 harvests can be obtained in a year. Sometimes, the whole plant is also harvested after about 6 months.

Post-harvest Processing

After harvesting, the plants are dried under shade for 3–4 days and stored in gunny bags.

Yield

Under favourable and well agro-managemental condition 2–2.5 tonnes per hectare of dry herb may be obtained.

Medicinal Properties

This bitter shrub is well-known under the name of kalmegh and forms the principal ingredient of a household medicine called *Alui*, which is extensively used in West Bengal. The extracted juice of the leaves, together with certain spices, such as cardamom, clove, cinnamon, etc. is dried in the sun, and made into little globules. This is prescribed for infants to relieve gripes, irregular bowel movement and loss of appetite.

The plant is very useful in case of general debility, dysentery and certain forms of dyspepsia.

The roots and the leaves are known as febrifuge, stomachic, tonic, alterative and anti-helminthic.

A saturated infusion of the whole plant in a dose of about half a pint, is used as a folk-medicine in fever.

Creat posses anti-typhoid and antibiotic properties. It is used to treat hepatic and digestive troubles. The decoction of the plant is used in some types of anaemia. In Thiland, the decoction of the dried leaves is used against high blood pressure.

4.8 Devil's Cotton (Syn. Perennial Indian Hemp)

Botanical Name

Ambroma augusta Linn.

Indian Name

Bengali & Gujarati–Olat-kambal; *Hindi*–Kumal, Sanukapashi, Ulatkambal; *Kannada*–Divvahatti, Melpundigida; *Orissi*–Chogowjai; Pisachogonjai; *Tamil*–Sivapputtutti; Assamis–Gunakhiakarai; Lepcha–Chuli.

Botanical Family

Sterculiaceae.

Suitable Places for Growing in India

It is found both wild and cultivated, throughout the hot and moisture parts of India from Punjab and Uttar Pradesh eastwards to Arunachal Pradesh, Assam, Meghalaya and Tripura, ascending to 1,200 m and southwards in peninsular India.

Botanical Description

Plant

A large, spreading, evergreen, quick–growing hairy shrub or small tree.

Stem

Branchlets, under side of leaves and inflorescence, soft-pubescent.

Leaves

Leaves membranous, finely acuminate; upper ovate or lanceolate, cordate, sometimes entire, about 6 inches long, short petioled; the lower orbicular-cordate, more or less lobed or angled, serrulate, in young plants upto 18 inches diametre; basal nerves 5–7, long petioled.

Flowers

Flowers in terminal or leaf-opposed, few-flowered cymes, peduncles extra-axillary with 2–3 large purple or dark-red centred bisexual flowers.

Calyx

Sepals 5, pale green, lanceolate, acute, 1 inch long, persistent.

Corrola

Petals 5, contorted in bud, claw concave in blooming, whitish and dark purple with purple hairs, ¼ inch long, terminating above in chocolate-coloured, elliptic appendages, 1 inch long.

Androecium

Staminal tube short, 5 petaloid larger, white and purple staminodes alternating with 5 sessile anthers.

Gynoecium

Styles 5, small, whitish, within the ring of staminodes.

Fruit

Fruit capsule, turbinate, membranous, 5-angled, winged, obtyramidal, septicidally 5-valved with truncate apex, 3.5–4.5 cm long.

Seeds

Seeds many, small, blackish, covered with silky hairs.

Species and Varieties

At present there is no named or certified varieties under this crop under cultivation.

Plant Parts Used

Whole plant.

Chemical Component

The root contains ambromine, choline, betaine, β-sitosterol, stigmasterol, friedelin, a basic compound picrate and a fixed oil.

The leaves contain taraxerol and its acetate, β-sitosterol-acetate, an aliphatic alcohol octacosanol, and probably a mixture of long chain fatty diols.

The stem-bark contains β-sitosterol and friedelin.

The presence of β-sitosterol and octacosane-1, 28-diol is reported in the heartwood.

The seeds contain a fixed oil (20.2 per cent) The fatty acid composition of the oil is as follows: palmitic (14.5 per cent), stearic (3.8 per cent), oleic (9.4 per cent), linoleic (71.5 per cent) and hexadecenoic (0.9 per cent)

Cultivation Procedure

Soil

The plant requires deep, fertile alluvial soils with good drainage facility.

Climatic Requirements

It is grown in all the tropical parts. Low winter temperature is not desirable which badly damages the plants.

Method of Propagation

Propagation can be done from seeds or from stem-cutting. Root-suckers are also sometimes used for propagation. The seeds loose viability quickly and hence, fresh seeds should be used. Germination is improved by soaking the seeds in water for 15 minutes at about 30°C. The optimum temperature for germination is 32°C.

About 24 kg of seed is required to pant in one hectare area of land.

The seeds are sown in the months of March–April in well-prepared nursery beds, which should be 8–10 cm raised from the ground level. Frequent and light sprinkling water as well as shading the nursery beds in hot-weather are necessary to protect the emerged seedlings.

Land Preparation

The field should be ploughed along with FYM to a fine tilth. Green manuring the field before planting is very effective.

Planting

The seeds can be sown either in nurseries for transplanting or directly in the field at a spacing of 2 m × 2 m.

When the seedlings are 15–20 cm tall, transplanting is done in the field.

Irrigation

Irrigation is required at least during the summer months, at weekly interval.

Intercultural Measures

The soil should be hoed at regular interval to control weeds. Ambroma field requires 2–3 weeding before the first crop is harvested.

Intercropping

The plants may be grown as an intercrop with any shrub or tree.

Crop Protection Measures

The plants are practically free from the attack of any serious pest or disease.

Harvesting

Harvesting of Fibre

Harvesting to secure fibre from the stem is done from July to December, i. e., 100–120 days after sowing, or after the growth of new stems following the previous harvest. For coarse fibre, the harvesting may be done as late as 6–7 months after sowing. The stems are cut 25 cm above the ground for new flush. Although upto four harvests can be done in a year, normally only two harvests are taken or sometimes only one.

Harvesting of Root

Roots are generally harvested from 2–3 year old plants. When freshly cut, the root produces a thick, gummy substances. The outer surface of the bark is dull brown and longitudinally wrinkled with small warty markings.

The inner surface of the root is whitish yellow and marked with fine longitudinal striatiars. The root bark is tasteless, slimy, odourless and tough, but not brittle.

Post-harvest Processing

Fibre

The fibre, extracted after retting the stem for 7–15 days is washed and beaten so as to make it supple and separate easily the individual strands. Over-drying is not desirable as it makes the fibre brittle.

Root

The thick roots are dug out by lifting the plants and then washed and cleaned. These are then sliced into suitable pieces and dried in sun or preferably in an incubator (below 40°C) and then these are stored in poly-bags.

The dry roots have brown and fibrous bark which is 0.5–1.0 mm thick. The thickness of the bark varies according to the ape and girth of the root.

Yield

Fibre

The yield of fibre greatly varies in accordance climatic, edaphic and other factors. An average yield of 735–990 kg is usually obtained from an hectare area of plantation.

Root

An average yield of 800–1000 kg root is usually obtained from an hectare area of plantation.

Medicinal Properties

The root is valued as an uterine tonic and an emmenagogue. It has a specific action on the female reproductive system and is used for treatment of dysmenorrhoea, infertility and other menstrual disorders. Powered roots act as abortifacient and anti-fertility agent and the petroleum-ether extract of the roots at a dose 50 mg/kg of body weight has been observed to have anti-implantation as well as abortifient properties in mice. The abortifacient activity was also noticed in extracts made with alcohol and chloroform extracts. The alcoholic extract made from the roots had shown acetylcholine-like action, comparable to that of choline or isolated smooth and skeletal muscles. The aqueous extract of the roots showed oxytocin action and has also been reported to possess galactotrophic effect on lactating albino rats.

The leaves are helpful in uterine disorders, diabetes, rheumatic pains of joints, and headche. The aqueous infusion of the fresh leaves and twigs made in cold condition is known to be demulcent and efficacious in gonorrhoea.

4.9 Fire Plant, (Syn. Officinal Leadwort, Rosy-Flowered Leadwort)

Botanical Name

Plumbago rosea Linn., (syn. *P. indica* Linn.)

Indian Name

Hindi–Chitra, Lal-chita, Rakta-chitra; *Bengali*–Lal-chita; *Marathi*–Lal-chitrak; *Gujarati*–Lal-chitrak, Rato-chatro; *Telugu*–Errachitramulam; *Kannada*–Kempacitramulam; *Orissi*–Rongachitamulo, Lalchita; *Tamil*–Cenkotiveli, Cithiramulam; *Malayali*–Chivappukoduveli.

Botanical Family

Plumbaginaceae.

Suitable Place for Growing in India

This plant may be grown throughout India in tropical region. It prefers moist and hot weather for its vigorous growth.

Botanical Description

Plant

Perennial herbs.

Stem

Stems herbaceous, erect, terete, slightly striate, simple, upward branching.

Roots

The root is cylindrical, sometimes irregularly bent or curved, 60–90 cm long and 1.3–2.0 cm thick, light yellowish brown, smooth, often with short transverse shallow fissures at the region of bends. Dried roots are darker or nearly black.

Leaves

Leaves alternate, membranous, entire, large, oblong, attenuate and slightly obtuse upwards, short-cuneate at the base, passing into a very short, amplexicaul, exauriculate petiole.

Flowers

Flowers rose-coloured, 3.5 cm long, forming very long terminal and axillary, lax spikes, which after flowering reach 30–60 cm; rachis quite glabrous. Bracteoles ovate-cuspidate, subequal, 4 times shorter than calyx, almost pellucid.

Calyx

Calyx red, short-cylindric, shortly and acutely 5-dentate, along the ribs covered with stipitate, bifarious and subsessile glands.

Corolla

Corolla hypocrateriform; corolla-tube slender, 4 times as long as the calyx, segments ovate, round, cuspidate.

Androecium

Stamen hypogynous, free from the corolla; filaments dilated at the base; anthers linear-oblong.

Gynoecium

Ovary free, one-celled, attenuated at the apex into a terminal filiform style which divides above into 5 longitudinally stigmatose branches.

Fruit

Capsule membranous, at length circumciss near the base, the decidus part often splitting into 5 valves from the base to the apex, fruit included within the calyx. Generally are not to be found to bear fruits in plains.

Seed

Seed filling the cell, pendulous from the apex of the funicle or more or less adnate to it, testa membranous; albumen farinaceous, copious, scanty.

Species and Varieties

A species having white flowers known as *P. zeylanica* is also cultivated in some places.

Plant Parts Used

Roots.

Chemical Component

The root bark of *P. indica* contains an orange yellow pigment named plumbagin (2-methyl-5-hydroxy-1, 4-naphthoquinone), a sitosterol glycoside, a sitosterol, a fatty alcohol, probably arachidyl alcohol, tannin, and an amorphous brown pigment. Plumbagin is the active principle of the drug, and is present in both *P. indica* and *P. zeylanica* up to the extent of about 0.9 per cent. The concentration of plumbagin varies according to the locality, growth and age of the plant, condition of the soil, and the season of the year. The older plant and drier soil the greater is the quantity of the active principle found in the root. The fresh roots give much higher yields of plumbagin than the roots stored for a long period.

The flowers contain 3-rhamnosides of pelargonidin, cyanidin, delphinidin and kaempferol.

Cultivation Procedure

Soil

Plumbago rosea can be grown successfully in sandy loam or light-red soils with good organic matter and drainage. A soil pH range of 7.5–8 is best for its good yield. It can also be grown in medium fertile soil with little care where other crops are unsuitable.

Climatic Requirements

This plant may be grown in tropical, moist and hot regions.

Method of Propagation

The plant is commercially propagated by vegetively by offsets or small cuttings and has never been known to be found in fruit. However, the offset cuttings can be rooted in polythene bags filled with the common pot mixture. The nursery can be raised during March and April. The cuttings are nursery planted in March–April will be ready for planting in the field by the end of May. The rooting efficiency can be increased by treating the cuttings with bio-fertilizer slurry. The cuttings should be dipped in the slurry prepared by mixing 5 g of *Azospirillum* sp. and 3 g of phosphobacteria in 100 ml water.

Land Preparation

The plant is usually grown in fields which are not well covered by irrigation systems. Mainly *Plumbago rosea* is grown in marginal fields where profitable crops can not be grown.

After receiving two to three showers the field is thoroughly pulverized by repeatedly ploughing, dishing or harrowing. Then the field is leveled and divided into plots of convenient sizes.

Planting

25–35 day-old seedlings attaining good height are transplanted in the field in 60 cm wide furrows at 60 cm apart.

Manuring

This crop does not require heavy doses of manure. However 250 kg of well-rotten FYM per hectare of land is a recommendation from the experts.

Irrigation

Light irrigation just after transplantation helps the seedlings for well establishment in the field. There is not any requirement of additional irrigation if there is good rainfal at regular intervals. But if there is a long dry season, life saving irrigation may be applied if required. Excessive rainfal is harmful.

Intercultural Measures

Weeding cum hoeing by hand at 25–30 days interval helps to control the weeds effectively and a better root growth.

Intercropping

The plants may be grown as an intercrop with *Eclipta alba* plantation.

Crop Protection Measures

P. indica is usually not attacked by pests and disease of serious nature.

Harvesting

Harvesting starts at 150 to 180 days after the transplanting. The entire plants are uprooted for roots, which are separated from aerial parts by cutting the stem 1–2 cm above the crown.

Post-harvest Processing

The uprooted roots are cut into smaller pieces of 7–10 cm to facilitate drying in the sun. The dried roots are then cleaned and trimmed before storing. The dry material should be stored in a cool and dry room, packed in gunny bag or boxes.

Precaustions need to be taken to avoid infestation with fungi and insects.

Yield

An average yield of about 5–6 q/ha of dried roots may be obtained from a well-managed commercial field.

Medicinal Properties

The root and root-bark are stomachic, carminative, astringent to the bowels, anthelmintic, alterative and cure intestinal troubles, dysentery, leucoderma, piles, bronchitis, itching, diseases of the liver, leprosy and other diseases.

In natural state, the bruised root of this plant is acrid and stimulating. When tempered with a little bland oil, it is used externally in rheumatic and paralytic affections.

The properties of the root have been stated by the old writers. O'shaughnessy first tried this drug to more than three hundred patents and found that the root-bark, being rubbed with water into a paste and applied to the skin, raised within 12–18 hrs.; and that it can be used as a cheap substitute for cantharides and cause no irritation of the genito-urinary organs.

In south India, the dried root is used as a remedy against secondary syphilis and leprosy.

The white juice is useful in eye troubles and as an external application against scabies. Its vesicating properties have been successfully utilized in curing some cases of leucoderma.

4.10 Garden Mint (Syn. Brown Mint, Lamb Mint, Mackerel Mint, Spearmint)

Botanical Name

Mentha viridis Linn, *M. spicata* Linn.

Indian Names

Hindi–Pahari Pudina; Ben.–Pudina; *Marathi*–Pudina.

Botanical Family

Labiatae.

Suitable Places for Growing in India

The plant can be cultivated throughout the plains of India successfully. It is widely grown in Uttar Pradesh, Madhya Pradesh, West Bengal, Orissa etc.

Botanical Description

Plant

Strong scented perennial herbs, 50 cm tall, root stock creeping, erect, aerial stolon leafy.

Stem

Stem short, branched, with short hair, dense.

Leaves

Leaves smooth, as the rest of the plant, or nearly so, sessile, lanceolate to oblong, acute, coarsely dentate, smooth above, glandular below.

Flowers

Flowers lilac, in loose, cylindrical, slender spikes, which are interrupted, with distant whorls; bracts awl-like, minute.

Calyx

Calyx campanulate; 5-toothed, throat of calyx naked.

Corolla

Corolla subequally 4-lobed, smooth.

Androecium

Stamens 4, equal, erect, distant, anther-cell parallel, dehiscing longitudinally.

Gynoecium

Ovary superior, deeply 4-lobed; style arms short, arise from the centre of the ovary between the lobes, erect, filiform, stigma 2-fid; ovules solitary in each lobe of the ovary, erect, anatropous.

Fruit

One seeded dry nutlets at the base of the calyx, smooth or reticulate.

Seeds

Seed solitary in nutlets, small, erect; albumen scanty or absent; embryo conform to the seed; radicle inferior.

Species and Varieties

The species is very variable and is considered to be a hybrid between *Mentha longifolia* and *M. rotundifolia*.

Mentha arvensis DC. var. *piperaecens* Holms. (Japanese mint), *Mentha piperita* Linn. (Pepper mint), *Mentha citrata* Ehrhart. (Lemon mint) are some species of Mint genus which are very similar to the Spearmint and can be cultivated similarly.

Plant Parts Used

Herbage, whole plant.

Chemical Component

The leaves have a characteristic, aromatic odour and a slightly pungent taste, not followed by a cooling sensation as in case of peppermint. Analysis of green leaves gave the following values: moisture (83.0 per cent); protein (4.8 per cent); fat (ether extract) (0.6 per cent); carbohydrates (8.0 per cent); fibre (2.0 per cent); and mineral matter (1.6 per cent); calcium–200 mg; phosphorus–80 mg; iron–15.6 mg; carotene (as vitamin A)–2,700 i.u.; nicotinic acid–0.4 mg; riboflavin–80 μg; and thiamine–50 μg/100 g; the leaves contain traces of copper (1.8 μg/g)

The fresh flowering herb on distillation yields 0.25-0.50 per cent of a volatile oil, known as Spearmint Oil. It is a colourless, yellow or greenish yellow liquid with the characteristic odour and taste of spearmint; the aroma improves on ageing.

The characteristic constituent of the oil is l-carvone. Oil distilled at Kanpur contained: carvone (55.8 per cent); terpenes (chiefly l-limonene and dipentene) (17.5 per cent); alcohol (as dihydrocarveol) (6.7 per cent); and esters (as dihydrocarveol acetate) (11.6 per cent) A sample of oil distilled from plants grown in Poona contained no carvone; a terpenic glyoxal was the principal constituent (54 per cent); other constituents of the oil were cineole (31.4 per cent) and traces of α-pinene, phellandrene and dihydrocarveol and its ester. The differences in the composition of oils are evidently due to varietal or even specific variations.

Cultivation Procedure

Soil

The plant grows well in rich, fertile soil with copious irrigation. It prefers well-drained, loamy, silty-loam to clayey-loam soils, well supplied with FYM and with a pH ranging between 6 and 7.

Climatic Requirements

A tropical climate with an annual rainfall of 100 cm is preferable for its vigorous growth. Light showers at planting time and ample sunshine at the time of harvest suit its cultivation. The stagnating water damages the crop and frost at the planting time are also not considered desirable.

Method of Propagation

Spearmint is mainly propagated by the use of stolons (underground stems) and these are transplanted during early spring.

Long stolons which 8–10 cm are collected from the old plantation during spring. The cuttings are soaked overnight in auxin (plant growth regulator) solution for better rooting.

Land Preparation

The land is repeatedly ploughed and brought to a fine tilth and weeds, stubbles and pebbles are to be removed. The field is divided into plots of convenient size and the soil is mixed with recommended dose of manures. About 20–25 tones of FYM is required for an hectare area of land. Groundnut cake, bone-meal, rapeseed cake and vermicompost are also beneficial for better growth of the plants. To remove mites and nematods from the field, prior application of neem cake is recommended at the doses of 7–12 kg/ha.

Planting

The rooted stolons are transplanted at 40–60 cm × 10–12 cm spacing in the field depending upon the soil fertility. About 250 kg of stolons are usually required to plant one hectare of land.

Manuring

In low fertile soil, 20–25 tonns of FYM/ha is recommended but in moderately fertile condition, the dose may be reduced at 15–18 tonns/ha. If irrigation facilities are available, it is recommended to green manure the field with leguminous crops. The seeds of the green manure crop may be treated with the bacterial inoculants before sowing so as to increase the development of root nodules which absorb atmospheric nitrogen and fix it into the soil.

Irrigation

The crop requires 12–15 irrigations during summer and 5–6 in autumn. Drainage is no doubt, an important factor. Intercultural Measures

The field requires intensive weeding at least during the early stages of growth for luxuriant growth of the plants.

Intercropping

The plants may be grown as an intercrop with Holy basil plantation.

Crop Protection Measures

In some areas the crop faces some attack from few pest and disease, which are as follows.

(1) *Termites and other Soil-borne Insect Attack*

Growing seedlings and young plants may be attacked by termites and other soil-borne insects. These may be effectively controlled by application of neem-cake or other neem-based biopesticides before planting.

(2) *Red Pumpkin Beetle (Radiopalpa foevicollis Lucas.) Attack*

The beetles feed on the growing young leaves. These may be effectively controlled by application of neem cake or other neem-based biopesticide before planting.

(3) *Caterpillars of Autographa nigrisigna Walk. Attack*

The caterpillars feed on the growing young leaves and cause small holes.

(4) *Stolon Rot Disease*

The plants are attacked by the *Macrophomina* fungi during rainy season.

The infected stolons show brown lesions which coalesce, turn black and result in necrosis.

(5) *Leaf Blight Disease*

Alternaria species attack the young and mature plants causing the disease.

(6) *Leaf Rust Disease*

During spring time *Puccinia menthae* Pers. attacks the young and mature leaves.

The rust disease may be avoided immerssing the stolon in hot water at 115°F before planting in field.

(7) *Leaf Rot Disease*

Young and mature leaves are affected by the fungus, *Rhizoctonia solani* Kuhn.

Harvesting

The first harvest is done before the onset of the rains after about 105 days of planting, particularly when the flower-buds begin to open. The fresh herbage at this stage contains 0.4–0.68 per cent of oil. The crop is cut 10 cm above the ground level on bright sunny days, since harvesting on cloudy or rainy day decrease the menthol content (with corresponding increase of methone) in the oil.

A second harvest is obtained after another 100 days in the month of October. The plant produces leaves for a number of years, but it is advisable to replant them annually in order to secure young and luxuriant growth.

Post-harvest Processing

The harvested crop is left in the fields for 2–4 hours for wilting to reduce its bulk before distillation. The stacking of the crop in heaps generates fermentation which might cause a heavy loss of oil.

Yield

The average yield is about 10 tonnes of fresh herbage per hectare per harvest, which, in turn, produces 80–100 l oil in a year.

Medicinal Properties

A volatile oil obtained from the plant is a well-known medicine for its antiseptic, antispasmodic, stimulant and carminative properties.

In Europe, the herb is considered a stimulant, stomachic, carminative and is used against nausea, flatulence, sickness, vomiting as well as an infant's cordial.

It's bruished fresh leaves, if applied, will relieve local pains and headache. A hot infusion, taken as tea, soothes stomach-ache, overcomes sickness and colicky diarrhoea. This is effective against menstrual colic.

4.11 Holy Basil (Syn. Mork's Basil, Rough Basil, Sacral Basil)

Botanical Name

Ocimum sanctum Linn.

Indian Names

Sanskrit–Ajaka, Brinda, Manjari, Parnasa, Patrapuspha, Suvasa Tulsi; *Hindi*–Tulsi, Baranda, Kala Tulsi; *Bengali*–Tulsi; *Marathi*–Tulasa, Tulasi Chajadha; *Gujarati*–Tulsi; *Telugu*–Tulasi, Brynda,

Gaggera, Krishna Tulsi, Nalla Tulsi; *Tamil*– Thulasi; *Kannada*– Vishnu Tulsi, Kari Tulsi, Sri Tulsi; *Malayali*–Trittavu.

Botanical Family

Labiatae.

Suitable Places for Growing in India

The plant can be successfully grown throughout India ascending up to 1,800 m in the Himalayas, and in Andaman and Nicobar Islands.

Botanical Description

Plant

Annual, 30–75 am high, much-branched.

Stem

Stems and branches usually purplish, sub quadrangular, sometimes woody below, clothed with soft spreading hairs.

Leaves

Leaves 2.5–5 by 1.6–3.2 cm, elliptic-oblong, obtuse or acute, entire or serrate, pubescent on both sides, minutely gland-dotted, base obtuse or acute, petioles 1.3–2.5 cm long, slender, hairy.

Flowers

Flowers in racemes 15–20 cm long in close whorls, bracts nearly 3 mm long and almost as broad as long, broadly ovate with a long slender acumen, ciliate, pedicels longer than the flowering calyx, slender, pubescent.

Calyx

Calyx campanulate, diflexed in fruit, 2-lipped, calyx 3–4 mm long in flower, pubesent, reaching 5 mm long in fruit, upper lip broadly obovate or sub-orbicular, much reflexed, very shortly apiculate; lower lip longer than the upper, the teeth lanceolate at the base, the 2 lateral with short straight, the 2 central with long slender awans which project beyond the upper lip and are much curved upwards.

Corolla

Corolla 2-lipped, tube short, not annulate within, upper lip subequally 4-fid; lower lip hardly longer than upper; declinate, entire, flat or nearly no; 4 mm long, purplish, upper lip pubecent on the back.

Androecium

Stamens 4, didynamous, declinate, exserted, filaments slender, the upper pair with a small bearded appendage at the base, lower pair connate bellow, naked; another-cells confluent, dehiscing longitudinally.

Gynoecium

Ovary superior, 4-partite, style simple from the centre of the ovary between the tubes, erect, filiform; stigma usually 2-fid; ovules solitary in each lobe of the ovary, erect, anatropous.

Fruit

Nutlets 1.25–1.5 mm long, broadly ellipsoid, nearly smooth, yellow with small black markings, mucilaginous when moistened, enclosed in the enlarged membranous veined strongly recurved calyx.

Seeds

Seed solitary in the nutlets, small, erect, albumen scanty; embryo conform to the seed; radicle inferior.

Species and Varieties

At present there are no named varities under this crop and only the types (*i*) Green Type (*i.e.* called "Sri Tulsi") and (*ii*) Purple Type (*i.e.* called " Krishna Tulsi") are under cultivation.

Plant Parts Used

Leaves, Seeds.

Chemical Component

On steam-distillation, the leaves produce a bright, yellow coloured volatile oil of pleasant aroma, which contains phenol, aldehyde, eugenol, eugenol methyl ether, carvacrol. The leaves also contain fairly high amount of ascorbic acid (83 mg/100 g) and carotene (2.5 mg/100 g).

The seeds of plant give a greenish yellow fixed oil (17.8 per cent) with good drying properties. The fatty acid composition of the oil is as follows–palmitic (6.9 per cent), stearic (2.1 per cent), oleic

(9.0 per cent), linoleic (66.1 per cent) and linolenic (15.7 per cent) The seeds contain a mucilage (hexouronic acid 27.2 per cent, pentoses 38.9 per cent and ash 0.2 per cent) which on hydrolysis yields xylose and acid polysaccharide.

Cultivation Procedure

Soil

The plant is quite hardy and can be grown on any type of soil except highly saline, alkaline or water-logged conditions. But sandy loam soil with good amount of organic matter is considered ideal.

Climatic Requirements

The crop has a wide adaptability and can be grown successfully in tropical and sub-tropical areas. Long days with high temperature are considered favourable for growth and oil content of plants.

Method of Propagation

The crop can be propagated from seeds or stem cuttings.

The nursery should be located preferably in partial shade with adequate irrigation facilities. Soil is to be tilled upto a depth of about 30 cm. Well rotten FYM (2 kg/sq m) is necessary to be applied to the soil and prepared to a fine tilth and seed beds of 4.5 × 1.0 × 0.2 m size are prepared. As the seeds are very small, the required quantity of seeds are mixed with sand in the ratio of 1: 4 and sown in nursery bed, 2 months before the onset of monsoon. They germinate in 8–12 days and seedlings become ready for transplanting in about 6 weeks when they produce 4–5 leaves.

Propagation can be done by terminal cuttings with about 90–100 percent success during October–December months. Cuttings with 8–10 nodes and 10–15 cm length are generally used. They are so prepared that except for the first 2–3 pairs of leaves the rest are trimmed off. Later, they are planted in the well prepared nursery beds or polythene bags. Within 4–6 weeks, the rooting is completed and they are ready for transplanting into the mainfield. Land Preparation

The land is repeatedly ploughed and brought to a fine tilth and weeds, stubbles and pebbles are to be removed. The field is divided into plots of convenient size and the soil is mixed with recommended dose of manures. About 20–25 tonnes of FYM is required for an hectare area of land. Groundnut cake, bone meal, rapeseed cake and vermicompost are also beneficial for better growth of the plants. To remove the mites and nematods from the field, prior application of neem cake is recommendate at the doses of 7–12 kg/ha.

Planting

The plants are transplanted at a spacing of 40 cm × 40 cm in the field.

Manuring

In the low fertile soil, 20–25 tonns of FYM/ha is recommended but in moderately fertile condition, the dose may be reduced at 15–18 tonns/ha. If irrigation facilities are available, it is recommended to green mannure the field with leguminous crops. The seeds of the green manure crop may be treated with the bacterial inoculants before sowing so as to increase the development of root nodules which absorb atmospheric nitrogen and fix it into the soil.

Irrigation

After transplanting, light irrigation is necessary to provide twice a week till one month so that the plants get well-established. Later, it is applied at weekly interval depending upon the rainfall and soil moisture condition.

Intercultural Measures

The first weeding should be done one month after planting and then after 30 days. Afterwards, no further weeding is required as the plants become bushy and cover the soil. After each harvest, weeding should be done to avoid weed growth in the interspaces.

Intercropping

The plants may be grown as an intercrop with Garden mint plantation.

Crop Protection Measures

(1) *Leaf Rollers Attack*

Both young and mature plants are affected by the pest.

(2) *Powdery Mildew Disease*

Young and mature plants are affected by this disease.

(3) *Seedling Blight Disease*

Seedlings in seedbed are generally effected by this disease.

Drainage should be ensured in the beds.

(4) *Root Rot Disease*

Seedlings at very young stage are affected by this disease.

Phytosanitory measures should be adopted to control the disease.

Harvesting

Harvesting should be done at full-bloom stage by cutting the plants at 15 cm from the ground level which ensures regeneration for subsequent harvests.

The first harvest is done after about 3 months of planting and subsequently, may be done at every 75 day interval. Harvesting should be done on bright sunny days to get good yield and oil of good quality.

Post-harvest Processing

Harvested plants are dried in sun for few hours and making into suitable pieces, these are stored in gunny bags.

Yield

The basil crop may yield about 10–15 tonns/ha of fresh herbage. As the herb contains about 0.1–0.23 per cent volatile oil, 10–23 litres of essential oil per hectare may be secured.

Medicinal Properties

The plant has stomachic, cholagogue, anthelmintic, alexiteric, antipyretic and other properties and is useful in diseases of the ear and blood, leucoderma, strangury, asthma, bronchitis, vomitting, lumbago, pains, hiccough, painful eye, purnlent discharge of the ear and may other aliments.

The decoction made from the roots is given as a diaphoretic in malarial fevers.

The leaves are effective expectorant and the leaf juice is used in respiratory troubles. The paste made from leaves is used in ringworm and other cutaneous diseases. An infusion made from the leaves is used as a stomachic in the gastric disorders of children and in hepatic disorders. Sometimes, the dried leaves are powered and employed as a snuff in ozaena. They are also effective to dislodge maggots. The juice instilled into the ear is said to be a good remedy for otic inflammations.

The seeds which are mucilaginous and demulant, are given in disorders of the genito-urinary tract.

In Sri Lanka, the herb is used in decoctions for cough and catarrh and sometimes chewed as a substitute for betel.

The fresh roots are ground and made into a paste with water and applied to the stings of wasps and bees besides bites of worms leeches etc.

4. 12 Indian Aloe (Syn. Barbados Aloe, Curacao Aloe, Tafarabad Aloe)

Botanical Name

Aloe barbadensis Mill.

Indian Names

Bengali & Sanskrit–Ghrita-kumari, Kanya; *Gujarati*–Kumarpathu, Kunawar; *Hindi*–Ghu-Kanwari, Ghi-Kuvar; *Kannada*–Kolasoare, Komarika, Maulisara; *Malayali*–Kattavazha; *Marathi*–Korphad; *Orissi*–Kumari, Mushaboro; *Tamil*–Bhottu-Katrazhae, Chirukattalai, Kottaalai; *Telugu*–Kalabanda, Chinna-kata-banda.

Botanical Family

Liliaceae.

Suitable Places for Growing in India

It is best suited for cultivation in arid and semi-arid region especially in Rajasthan, Gujarat, Madhya Pradesh, Maharastra, Karanataka, Tamil Nadu, Kerala, Andhra Pradesh.

Botanical Description

Plant

Plant coarse-looking, perennial, shallow-rooted plant with a short stem. The plant generally grows close to the ground in a typical rosette shape. The plants have multiple tuberous roots and many supporting roots penetrating into the soil.

Stem

Aloe does not have a true stem. The leaves are originated on a stalk like stem of 30–60 cm height.

Leaves

The fleshy leaves about 60 cm long, 10 cm broad and 1.5– 2 cm thick are densely crowded, strongly cuticularized and have a spiny margin with thin-walled, tabular cells.

Flowers

Scapes longer than the leaves, scaly, branched racemes long, dense, bracts short-lanceolate, membranous, longer than the short pedicle. Flowers pendulous, imbricate, yellow, actinomorphic, vary from yellow to rich orange in colour and are arranged in auxillary spikes.

Perienth

Perienth in two whorls of 3 calyx each, perienth segment united into a cylindric or companulate straight or slightly curved tube, tips sometimes free, imbricate in bud.

Androecium

Stamens 6 in two whorls, outer whorl having longer flaments than inner whorl, filaments inserted into a pit in the connective; anthers linear, dorsifixed, usually dehiscing longitudinally, somewhat excerted. Most of the species are made sterile with scaecely any fertile pollen.

Gynoecium

Ovary 3-celled, superior; ovules 2 or more from the inner angles of the cells, anatropous, axile placentation; style usually simple, often long.

Fruit

Fruit loculicidal capsul, usually 3-celled.

Seeds

Aloe does not produce viable seeds inside the pods.

Species and Varieties

The following species are cultivated in many places of India.

1. *Aloe vera* var. *chinensis* Baker (Deccan Area)
2. *A. vera* var. *littoralis* Koening ex. Baker (Madras to Rameswaram)
3. *A. abyssinica* Linn. (Kathiawar coast)
4. *A. variegata* Linn. (Maharastra)
5. *A. ferox*
6. *A. perryi*
7. *A. africana*
8. *A. spicata*

In trials conducted at the National Bureau of plant Genetic Resources, New Delhi, the aloe accessions IC-111271, IC-111280, IC-111269, IC-111273, IC-111279 and IC-111267 are reported to contain high aloin contents and the accessions, IC-111267, IC-1112660, IC-111280, IC-111277, high gel contents.

Plant Parts Used

Leaves.

Chemical Component

Aloe contains cathartic anthraglycosides as its active principles, these are mostly C-glucosides, notably barbaloin, which is a glucoside of aloe emodin. The concentration of these glucosides vary from the types of aloe ranging from 4.5 to 25 per cent of aloin. Other constituent, present include aloesin and its aglycone aloesone (a chromone), free anthraquinones (e.g aloe emodin) and resins. The mucilage of the leaves contains glucose, galactose, mannose and galacturonic acid, in addition to an unidentified aldopentose and a protein (0.013 per cent) with 18 amino acids. The palnt contains aloesone and aloesin and aloe-lectins.

The plant produces at least 6 antiseptic agents such as lupeol, salicylic acid, urea nitrogen, cinnamonic acid, phenols and sulphur. It contains at least three anti-inflammatory fatty acids, cholesterol, campersterol and β-sitosterol. Aloe also contains 23 polypeptides in its juice.

Cultivation Procedure

Soil

Aloe is a hardy plant and grows on a variety of soils. It is grown successfully in marginal to sub-marginal soils having low fertility. The plants have tendency to tolerate high pH with high sodium and potassium salts. However, it is observed that its growth is faster under medium fertile, heavier soils such as black cotton soils of central India, though well-drained loam to coarse sandy loam soils with moderate fertility and pH upto 8.5 are preferred for its commercial cultivation. Water-logged conditions and problematic soils do not suit the palnts.

Climatic Requirements

It is grown in almost all parts in India, even under constant drought condition. However, the crop grows well in entire tropical and sub-tropical regions. It is usually cultivated between March and June and is found growing in warm, humid or dry climate with even 150–200 cm to about 35–40 cm of yearly rainfall during growing period. However, in dry regions, the crop should be provided with protective irrigation for better yield.

Method of Propagation

For propagation of the plants, root suckers are preferred but cuttings from rhizomes may also be used as planting materials. About 3–4 months old suckers having 4–5 leaves and 20–25 cm in length are used.

Land Preparation

Deep ploughing is not required as roots of aloe do not reach below 20–30 cm. Depending upon the soil type and agro-climatic condition, 1–2 ploughings followed by leveling may be done. The field should be cleaned thoroughly of weeds and if required, small channels may be prepared for drainage. About 25 t/ha of FYM is also added. Field may be divided into suitable sized plots (10–15m × 3m) considering the slope and source of irrigation available.

Planting

Suckers should be planted during monsoon to get better field survival and subsequent growth of the plants. However, under irrigated condition, planting may be done around the year except in winter months (November to February)

Suckers are planted in about 15 cm deep pits made just at the time of planting at 60 × 60 cm or 60 × 45 cm apart. The suckers should be planted in such a way that two-third portion of the sucker should be under the ground.

After planting of suckers, the soil around the root zone must be firmly pressed and drainage must be made to avoid water stagnation.

About 28,000–34,000 suckers are needed for planting in a hectare area of land.

Manuring

In general, the crop responds well to application of FYM or compost. About 10–15 tonnes of the manure may be applied at the time of soil preparation and also in subsequent years. But it is not a common practice since the crop is cultivated in marginal and sub-marginal lands. If sufficient quantity of wood-ash is available, that can be applied in the pits at the time of planting. It helps in establishment of plants and their subsequent growth.

Irrigation

The crop has the ability to withstand water-stress but to get higher yield, irrigation at critical stages of growth is advisable.

First irrigation should be given just after planting of suckers followed by 2–3 irrigations till plants get established. However, 4–6 irrigations per year may be enough for proper growth of the plants.

After each picking of leaves, light irrigation may be given depending upon the availability of water. Water should not be allowed to stagnate near the plant.

Intercultural Measures

The field should be made free from weeds throughout the growing period of the crop. 2–3 hand weedings followed by light hoeing per year promote growth and suckering. First weeding and hoeing should be completed within a month after planting. However, in subsequent years, two weeding with light hoeing in each year found to be sufficient to minimize the weed population in the field. Unproductive and diseased plants as well as dried flower stalks should be removed regularly.

Intercropping

During the first year of planting, more than 40 per cent land remains unutilized. Thus, attempt should be made to utilize the field in efficient manner. For this purpose, suitable leguminous or less competitive intercrops, like cluster bean, groundnut, seasame, isabgol, coriander, cumin etc. could be grown successfully in the inter-spaces under arid and semi-arid condition that can generate additional income. Besides that, the soil condition will also improve with leguminous crops. From second year onwards, such crops may not be encouraged otherwise foliage yield and quality of the produce will be adversely affected.

Crop Protection Measures

Normally, the plant is not affected by any pest and disease of a serious nature. But recently the following pests and diseases have been reported from some parts of the country, such as,

Leaf Spot Diseases

Altarnaria alternata and *Fusarium solani* attack the young and mature plants especially during rainy season.

Mealy Bug Attack

Wrapping the stem with polythene prevents crawling of the bugs.

Termite Attack

Growing seedlings and young plants may be attacked by termites and other soil-borne insects. These may be effectively controlled by application of neem-cake or other neem-based biopesticides before planting.

Harvesting

An aloe plantation gives commercial yield from second year to fifth year of planting and the first crop may be harvested after eight months. Generally, 3–4 pickings per year can be taken up depending upon the growth of plants.

While harvesting, the plants can be removed manually or with the help of a tractor drawn dise harrow or cultivator. The broken rhizome part left in the soil throws out new sprouts in spring for raising the succeeding crop. After fifth year of harvesting, the crop needs replanting.

Post-harvest Processing

Freshly harvested leaves are marketed as soon as possible.

Yield

On an average, 15–20 tonns/ha fresh leaves are obtained from second year of plantation. However, well-managed irrigated crop can give fresh leaves of upto 35 tonns/ha.

Medicinal Properties

The plant produces at least 6 antiseptic substances such as lupeol, salicylic acid, urea, nitrogen, cinnamonic acid, phenols and sulphur. All these substances are recognised as antiseptics because they kill or control mold, bacteria, fungus and viruses. Lupeol and salicylic acid present in the juice are two very effective pain killer.

Aloe contains at least three anti-inflammatory fatty acids, cholesterol, campersterol and β-sitosterol (plants sterols) These are highly effective in treatment for burns, cut, scrapes, abrasions, allergic reactions, rheumatoid arthritis, rheumatic fever, acid indigestion, ulcers, and many inflammatory conditions of the digestive system and other internal organs, including the stomach, small intestine, colon, liver, kidney and pancreas. β-sitosterol is also a powerful anti-cholestromatic which helps to lower harmful cholesterol levels.

About 23 polypeptides (immune stimulators) are present in aloe juice which helps to control a broad spectrum of immune system diseases and disorders.

The phypeptides and anti-tumor agent, i. e., aloe emodin and aloe lectins, are now used in the treatment of cancer.

Aloe is widely used in menstrual diseases, stomach pain, after pregnancy tonic etc. but not prescribed to expectant women. It is also used in pelvic congestion and uterine disorders with iron and carmin. Aloe roots is used in colic pain. Aloe mucilage are used in painful inflammation and the pulp keeps the nervous system under control if applied on head.

Various preparations from aloe extraction, juice, polysaccaride, stabilized gel etc. are prepared for tropical use in burns, insect and fish bites, skin ailments, arthritis, myopathies, cosmetics etc.

Fresh leaf is eaten to alleviate cold and with salt it keeps blood in good condition and relieves constipation.

Anti-inflammatory composition containing aloe extract and steroids, glycoprotein, alocutin A from aloe may be used for cancer and skin diseases.

4.13 Indian Pennywort, (Syn. Thick-leaved Pennywort)

Botanical Name

Centella asiatica Urban.

Indian Names

Bengali–Thankuni; *Gujarati*–Moti Brahmi; *Hindi*–Brahma-manduki, Brahmibooti, Khulakhudi, Mandookaparni; *Kannada*–Brahmisoppu, Vandelaga-illikiwigidda; *Malayali*–Kodangal, Muyalchevi; *Marathi*–Karinga, Karivana; *Orissi*–Thalkudi; *Sanskrit*–Mandukaparni, Mutthil, Brahmamanduki; *Tamil*–Vallarai; *Telugu*–Brahmi, Saraswataku; *Assamis*–Manimuni; *Meghalayan*–Bat-maina; Tri.–Thankuni, Thunimankuni.

Botanical Family

Umbelliferae, Apiaceae.

Suitable Places for Growing in India

Throughout the tropical parts of India, this plant is commonly found as a weed in crop fields and other waste places up to an altitude of 600 m.

Botanical Description

Plant

A prostrate, faintly aromatic, stoloniferous perennial herb, up to 2 m. long.

Stem

Stem glabrous, long, pink and striated, filiform, rooting at the nodes, internode long, schizogenous oil ducts present in the stem, roots and mostly also among the mericarps; these are known as *'vittae'*.

Leaves

Leaves 1.3–6.3 cm diam., several from the rootstock which often have much elongated petioles, and 1–3 from each node of the stems, orbicular–reniform, rather broader them long, more or less cupped, entire or shallowly crenate-dentate, glabrous on the upper surface and sparsely hairy on the lower, with numerous slender nerves from a deeply cordate base; petioles very variable in length 7.5–15 cm long or more, channeled, glabrous or nearly so; stipule short, adnate to the petioles forming sheathing base.

Flower

Flowers in fascicled umbel, each umbel consisting of 3–4 pink or white, sessile (rarely pedicelled), small, bisexual, regular, epigynous flowers; peduncles pubescent or glabrous, short, pink; bracts ovate, acute, concave, 2 beneath each umbel.

Calyx

Sepals 5, free, often scarcely indicated.

Corolla

Petals 5, free, often unequal, with short claws, imbricate.

Androecium

Stamens 5, free, alternating with petals and arising from an epigynous disc.

Gynoecium

Carpels-2, median, mostly prominently ribbed and often with parallel resinous canal; style-2, free but swollen at the base to form a stylopodium; ovary inserted on a disc, inferior, ovary 2-celled with one pendulous ovule in each cell; stigma bifid.

Fruit

Cremocarp 4 mm long, longer than broad, ovoid, oblong, woody, hard, dull brown, laterally compressed, with thickened pericarp, reticulate-rugose, often crowed by the persistant petals, the primary and secondary ridges distinct.

Seed

Seed one in each carpel, pendulous from the point of attachment to the carpophore; testa thin; albuminous with minute embryo, straight, near the apex of the seed; radical superior.

Species and Varieties

At present there is no named or certified varieties under this crop under cultivation.

Plant Parts Used

Leaves, whole plant.

Chemical Component

The leaves are rich in carotenoids, vitamin B and C. The flavonoids, 3-glucosylquercetin, 3-glucosyl kaempferol and 7-glucosyl kaempferol have been isolated from the leaves.

Analysis of leaves gave the following values: moisture (87.2 per cent), protein (1.7 per cent), fat (0.7 per cent), carbohydrate (4.8 per cent), crude fibre (3.4 per cent), and ash (2.3 per cent), calcium–176.0 mg/100 g, phosphorus–72.0 mg/100 g, iron–12.0 mg/100 g, vitamin C –42.0 mg/100 g, niacin–0.8 mg/100 g, carotene–2400 μg/100 g, energy–32.0 kcal/100g.

An ethanolic extract (80 per cent) of the plant showed the presence of a number of free amino-acids.

Two glycosides, asiaticoside and madecassoside have been isolated from the plant grown in Malagasy. On hydrolysis, those glycosides yield the triterpene acids, asiatic acid and madegascaric acid (madecassic acid) respectively. These acids are also present in free form in the plant. A sample of the air-dried plant from Sri Lanka showed the presence of three triterpene acids, *viz.* centic, centellic and centoic and a water soluble glycoside, centelloside which, on hydrolysis, gives centellic acid. The triterpene acids and glycosides isolated from the Sri Lankan plant are different from those isolated from the Malagasy variety of the plant.

Samples of the Indian plants collected from different places showed the presence of the following glycosides: indocentelloside, brahmoside, brahminoside, asiaticoside, thakuniside and isothankuniside.

The corresponding triterpene acids obtained on hydrolysis of the glycosides are: indocentoic, brahmic, asiatic, thankunic and isothankunic. These acids except the last two are also present in free form in the plant besides isobrahmic and betulic acid. Presence of mesoinositol, a new oligosaccharide, "centellose", kaempferol, quercetin and stigmasterol has also been reported. Indocentoic acid is isomeric with centoic acid present in the Sri Lankan plant. The variation in the chemical composition of Indian samples of the plant is attributed to geographical conditions.

An alcoholic extract of the herb gave an essential oil possessing the strong odour of the herb, a fatty oil, tannin and a resinous substance. The major terpenoidal constituents identified in the ether extract of the herb are β-caryophyllene, trans-β-farnesene, germacrene-D and an unidentified terpenic acetate. Presence of sitosterol, stigmasterol and campesterol is also reported. The fatty oil consists of the glycerides of palmitic, stearic, lignoceric, oleic, linoleic and linolenic acids. An alkaloid, hydrocotylin has been isolated from the dried plant. A bitter principle, vellarine and pectic acid are present in the leaves and roots.

Asiaticoside is useful in the treatment of leprosy and certain types of tuberculosis. Madecassol, an extract of the plant containing madecassic acid, asiatic acid and agiaticoside accelerates cicatrization and grafting of wounds. Madecassoside and madecassic acid also show anti-inflammatory activity.

Cultivation Procedure

Soil

The plant is found in abundance on moist, sandy or clayey soils, often in large clumps forming a dense green carpet.

Climatic Requirements

The plants are propagated vegetatively by runners and clumps, but seeds can also be used. Runner cuttings about 3–5 cm long, each containing few leaves, nodes and roots are ideal planting materials. These can be obtained by cutting mother plants into small pieces with roots.

Land Preparation

The land is prepared by repeated ploughing and leveling to bring to a fine tilth. About 25 tonns of FYM per hectare is mixed well with the soil at the time of the last ploughing. The land is laid out into plots of convenient sizes with provision of irrigation channels for easy management.

The land should be irrigated a day before planting for successful establishment of plant cuttings.

Planting

The cuttings are transplanted in wet soil at a spacing of 40 cm × 40 cm. Heavy irrigation should be done immediately after planting. Ideally, the plants should be transplanted in March–June and are allowed to grow and proliferate through hot and humid months of the monsoon till September, after which harvesting may be done.

Manuring

Thankuni responds well to the application of well-decomposed FYM @ 15–20 tonnes per hectare area of land at the time of field preparation.

Irrigation

Immediately after transplanting, irrigation is essential for successful survival of the plants. Subsequently, the fields are irrigated by flooding as per requirement usually at every 7–8 days.

Intercultural Measures

Initially, hand-weeding is required at every 5–20 days interval. Later, as the plant proliferates and form a dense mat of vegetation, weeding may be done sporadically as and when needed.

Crop Protection Measures

Thankuni is usually not attacked by pests and diseases of serious nature.

Harvesting

The leaves, stems and roots may be harvested after two months of plantation.

They can be ideally harvested by cutting in such a way so that the upper portion of the stem 4–5 cm from the base are removed and rest left for subsequent regeneration.

Leaves may be harvested 6–8 times in year.

Post-harvest Processing

The plants can be dried in a conventional manner by spreading on the ground in open sun or partial shade. Alternatively, they can be dried at 80°C in hot-air-oven for 30 minutes immediately after harvest. After this, they can be further air-dried by spreading on the ground at room temperature or in the oven at 37°C.

The dry material should be cleaned and made free from any external matter. The dry material should be stored in a cool and dry room, packed in gunny bag or boxes, having concrete flooring and away from walls.

Precautions need to be taken to avoid infestation with fungi and insects.

Yield

Under favourable condition 3–3.5 tonns per hectare of dry herb may be obtained.

Medicinal Properties

The plant is acrid, bitter, sweet, digestible, laxative, cooling, tonic, alterative, alexiteric, antipyretic; improves appetite, voice, memory cures leucoderma, anaemia, urinary discharges, diseases of the blood, bronchitis, inflammations, fevers, "kapha", biliousness, enlargement of spleen, thirst, asthma, smallpox and is used in insanity.

The plant is a useful alterative and tonic in diseases of skin, nerves and blood. In some parts of India, the people are in the habit of taking the powdered dried leaves with milk for improving their memory and as an alterative tonic.

The plant is used for treatment of leprosy and skin diseases and also to improve memory. In pharmacological and clinical trials it has been found to improve the power of concentration and general ability and behaviour of mentally retarded children. The plant is known to be effective in cholera. A cold poultice of the fresh herb is used as an external application in rheumatism, elephantiasis and hydrocele. For treating leprosy and other skin diseases it is used making ointment or as a dusting power. Compound proprietary preparations of the plant have been patented for cosmetic use in France. Internally it is used as a tonic and used in bronchitis, asthma, gastric catarrh, leucorrhoea, kindney troubles, urethritis and dropsy. A decoction of very young shoots is given for haemorrhoids.

The plant is efficacious in peptic ulcers. It is one of the components of the drug "Geriforte" which is used for senile pruritus. A paste of the plant is applied on boils and tumours. The whole plant mixed with *Drymaria cordata* Wild and *Oxalis corniculata* Linn. is boiled and taken to cure dysentery. In large doses the plant acts as narcotic, producing cephalagia, vertigo and sometimes coma. The plant is also considered as aphrodisiac and used in renal diseases.

Juice of the leaves with ginger and black paper is taken for cough. Leaf juice with palm jaggery is given to women as a tonic after delivery. It is rubbed on the forehead to cure severe headache. Mixed with bath water, the juice of leaves is used in eczema. The leaf extract is used in the preparation of a medicated oil for fracture bone.

4.14 Indian Privet (Syn. Five Lipped Chasti Tree)

Botanical Name

Vitex negundo Linn.

Indian Names

Hindi–Sambhalu, Shambalu, Shivari, Nisinda; *Bengali*–Nisinda, Samalu, Nirgundi; *Marathi*–Nirgundi, Nisind, Nigudi; *Gujarati*–Nagoda, Nagaol; *Telugu*–Vaavili, Tellavaaviti; *Tamil*–Vellai-nocohi, Nirkkundi, Venmochi; *Kannada*–Lakkigida, Nakkilu, Nekki; *Malayali*–Vellanocchi; *Orissi*–Beyguna, Begundia, Nirgundi; *Punjabi*–Banna, Marwan, Shwari; *Assamis*–Pasutia, Aggla-chita.

Botanical Family

Verbenaceae.

Suitable Places for Growing in India

This shrub is very common in tropical and sub-tropical India. It can be successfully cultivated on waste lands upto 1500 m of height. It is abundant along the banks of rivers, in moist situation, open waste lands and near the deciduous forests.

Botanical Description

Plant

A large shrub or sometimes a small slender tree.

Stem

Stem erect, bark thin, grey; branchlets quadrangular, whitish with a fine tomentum.

Leaves

Leaves 3–5 foliate; leaflets lanceolate, acute, the terminal leaflet 5–10 by 1.6–3.2 cm with a petiolule 1–1.3 cm long, the lateral leaflets smaller with a very short petiolule, all nearly glabrous above, covered with a fine white tomentum beneath, base acute; common petioles 2.5–3.8 cm long.

Flower

Flowers in pedunculate branched tomentose cymes, opposite along the quadrangular tomentose rhachis of a large terminal often compound pyramidal panicle (axilary peduncles in the upper axils sometimes present); bracts 1.5–2.5 mm long, laceolate, caducous.

Calyx

Clyx 3 mm long, white-tomentose; teeth 2, triangular, 0.8–1 mm long.

Corolla

Corolla companulate, truncate or shortly 5 toothed, corolla 1 cm long, bluish purple, tomentose outside, hairy inside at the insertion of the stamens; upper lip 2 mm long, divided to the base into 2 obtuse lobes; lower lip large, 5 mm long, with 2 short oblong obtuse, lateral lobes 1.5 mm deep, and a large broadly obovate, crenulate terminal lobe, 4 mm long.

Androecium

Stamens 4, didynamous, usually exserted; filaments hairy at the very base; anther-cells at first paralled and pendulous, afterwards divaricate, often twisting so that the lower ends are erect.

Gynoecium

Ovary 2-celled, glabrous; style glabrous; filiform; stigma 2 forked; ovules 4.

Fruit

Fruit ovoid drup less than 5–6 mm diam., black when ripe; invested at the base by the somewhat enlarged calyx; endocarp bony, normally 4-celled and 4-seeded, but some of the cells often suppressed.

Seed

Seeds obovate or oblong, exalbuminous; embryo straight; radicle inferior.

Plant Parts Used

Leaves, roots stem-bark.

Chemical Component

A greenish-yellow oil is obtained on steam-distillation of fresh leaves. Besides that, the leaves also contain aldehydes and ketone (22.5 per cent), phenolic derivatives (15 per cent), cineol (10 per cent), alkaloids, nishindine, hydrocotylene, glucononitol, *p*-hydroxybenzoic acid, glucoside, tannic acid, vitamin C (150 mg/

100 g on fresh weight basis), carotene (3,500 µg/100 g on fresh weight basis), 5-hydroxyisophthalic acid, 3-4 dihydroxybenzoic acid, aucubin, agnuside, casticin, orientin, isoorientin etc.

Cultivation Procedure

Soil

The crop thrives well on variety of soils but is largely grown in sandy loam, loam and red lateritic soil. In many places, it is grown along river banks and in sloppy land and also as a hedge-plant. The plant cannot does not grow well under water-logged situation.

Climatic Requirements

The plant thrives well in tropical and subtropical climates but the growth in tropical situation is better. It prefers warm and moist condition all round the year and where rainfall is high and well distributed, it can be grown as a rainfed crop. The plants may be successfully grown upto an elevating of 1,050 m.

Method of Propagation

Vitex negundo can be propagated from one year old stem-cutting during rainy-season.

Stem cuttings obtained from lateral stems are generally used. Lateral stems which are one year old and of pencil thickness are suitable materials for rooting. Pre-soaking the cuttings overnight in 25–60 ppm NAA solution results in better rooting.

Land Preparation

The land is repeatedly ploughed and brought to a fine tilth and weeds, stubbles and pebbles are to be removed. The field is divided into plots of convenient size and the soil is mixed with recommended dose of manures. About 20–25 tones of FYM is required for an hectare area of land. Groundnut cake, bone-meal, rapeseed cake and vermicompost are also beneficial for better growth of the plants. To remove mites and nematods from the field, prior application of neem cake is recommended at the doses of 7–12 kg/ha.

Planting

Well-rooted and healthy cuttings are planted in the field at the beginning of rainy season at a spacing of 100 cm × 50 cm.

Manuring

In low fertile soil, 20–25 tonns of FYM/ha is recommended but in moderately fertile condition, the dose may be reduced at 15–18 tonns/ha. If irrigation facilities are available, it is recommended to green manure the field with leguminous crops. The seeds of the green manure crop may be treated with the bacterial inoculants before sowing so as to increase the development of root nodules which absorb atmospheric nitrogen and fix it into the soil.

Irrigation

The plants are drought-resistant and do not require much water. Also, a majority of the growers raise a rain-fed crop during the monsoon season. Light irrigations are required in case of inadequate rains. The irrigated crop requires 5–6 light irrigations.

Intercultural Measures

The crop is given 2–3 periodic hoeing and weeding at 20 or 30 days interval or as per requirement. Mulching with rice straw or cut–grass is recommended to minimise weed growth

At early flowering stage, the top 2 cm portions of the plant are removed to promote vegetative growth and alkaloid content.

Intercropping

The plants can be grown as intercrop with *Phyllantus emblica, Solanum nigram* etc.

Crop Protection Measures

Vitex is a hardy crop in nature and is free from any pest and diseases of serious nature.

Harvesting

Leaves may be plucked after 6 months of planting and may be repeated at interval of 5–6 months.

Root and stem bark may be collected after 3–4 months of planting.

Post-harvest Processing

Leaves

Leaves are collected in sunny day and dried in shade. The dried leaves are stored in gunny bags in dry places.

Roots

The roots are dug out and then washed in clean water. They are then made into suitable pieces and dried in sun or preferably in an incubator (40°C) after which they are stored in gunny bags.

Stem-bark

The stem-bark is stripped off, washed and properly cleaned. They are then sliced into suitable pieces and dried in sun or preferably in an incubator (40°C) and are stored in gunny bags.

Yield

The yield of leaves may be 2–3 tonnes/ha. Roots may be obtained 4–5 tonnes and stem-bark 1–1.5 tonnes/ha.

Medicinal Properties

The plant has stomachic and anthelmintic properties. It promotes the growth of hair and useful in diseases of the eye, consumption, inflammations, leucoderma, enlargement of the spleen, bronchitis, asthma, biliousness, painful teething of children etc. The root is an antidote of snake-venom. It is also considered as a tonic, febrifuge and expectorant.

The aromatic leaves are vermifuge and a decoction of Vitex leaves with addition of long pepper is prescribed in catarrhal fever with heaviness of head and dullness of hearing. For relief from headache, a pillow stuffed with the leaves of the plant is placed under the head. The sap of the leaves is effective in removing foetid discharges and worms from ulcers. An oil made with the leaves is applied in sinus pain and scrofulous sores.

The leaves are discutient and are useful to remove swelling of the joints from acute rheumatism and of the testes from suppressed gonorrhoea. In the Konkan region, the leaf juice along with maka (*Eclipta alba*), tulsi (*Ocimum sanctum*) and ajwan seeds is brinsed, steeped and given in doses of six massas in rheumatism.

The decoction made from the leaves is used as a bath in the puerperal state of women in many places. In Karnataka, the people are in the habit of treating febrile, catarrhal and rheumatic affections by means of a vapour-bath, prepared from this plant.

The dried leaves are smoked as a relief against headache and catarrh. The dried fruits serve as vermifuge.

In Sri Lanka, the leaves, bark and roots are used for toothache, rheumatism, eye diseases and as a carminative and vermifuge.

The flowers are used in fever, diarrhoea and hepatitis. The fruits have analgesic properties and are valued as medicine in China.

4.15 Indian Senna (Syn. Tinnevelly Senna)

Botanical Name

Cassia angustifolia Vahl.

Indian Names

Sanskrit–Bhumiari, Bhupadma, Svarnapatri; *Hindi*–Hindi-sana, Sanay Sana Ka Patt, *Tamil*–Nilavira, Nelavakai; Guj–Nat-ki-sana; Beng–Sanna-makki, Son-pat; *Marathi*–Shona-makhi; *Telugu*–Nela-tangedu; *Kannada*–Nnelavarike; *Malayali* –Nila Vaka

Botanical Family

Caesalpineae.

Suitable Places for Growing in India

It is cultivated commercially in Gujarat, Rajasthan and Tamil Nadu. In Tamil Nadu, it is cultivated in the districts of Tirunelveli, Ramanathapuram, Madurai, Salem and Tiruchirapalli etc.

Botanical Description

Plant

Shrub or undershrub with pale suterete or obtusely angled erect or ascending branches, below 1 mt in height.

Stem

Stem erect, stout, glabrous, much branched.

Leaves

Leaves abruptly pinnate, usually 5-8 jugate, leaflets oval-lanceolate; glabrous.

Flowers

Flowers yellow, in axillary racemes, erect, laxly many-flowered, usually considerably exceeding the subtending leaf Bract, membranous, ovate or obovate, caducous.

Calyx

Calyx deeply divided, tube very short, segments 5, imbricate, obtuse, membranous, Legume flat, 15–17 mm in breath.

Corolla

Petals 5, imbricate, subequal or the lower the largest.

Androecium

Stamens 10, fertile stamen 7, the other reduced to staminodia, anthers uniform or those of the lower stames the larger, dehiscing by terminal pores.

Gynoecium

Ovary superior, free at the bottom of the calyx, ovules many, style short stigma terminal.

Fruit

Pods less than 30 cm long, more or less flattened, usually septale between the seeds dehiscent or indehiscent.

Seeds

Seeds horizontally compressed, albuminous, obovate, cuneate, cotyledons plane.

Species and Varieties

Cassia acutifolia Del., *C. obovate, C. italica,C. aborata* etc. are other species which are cultivated many places of India.

alft–2, Sona, Tinnervelly Senna are some famous high yielding varieties of *Cassia anguistifola.*

Plant Parts Used

Leaves, Pods.

Chemical Component

The cathartic principles of senna are soluble in water and dilute alcohol but insoluble in absolute alcohol. The odorous and colouring principles are soluble both in alcohol and water. From the leaf powder left after extraction with petrol ether, flavonol and anthraquinone groups of compounds separately may be obtained. The flavonol portion consists of *iso*rhamnetin and kaempferol in more or less equal quantities, while the anthraquinone portion contains mostly rhein along with small quantities of emodin.

A new crystalline compound $C_{15}H_{18}O_9$ insoluble in ether and sparingly soluble in water, has been isolated. The compound is phenolic in nature and has not been identified. The presence of glycosides one easily hydrolysable yielding emodin and activity cathartic, and the other hydrolysable with difficulty, and slow in laxative effect. 2 glycosides were isolated, *viz.*, sennoside A and sennoside B which are believed to be the laxative principles of senna, both having the same formula, C21H20O10, but differing principally in the manner of linkage of glucose to the aglycone fraction. Among other substances reported from time to time as being present in senna are: mannitol, sodium potassium phonic acid, an ethereal oil and a resin. The flowers contain chrysophanic acid. The occurrence of oxymethyl anthraquinone in the fruit to the extent of 1.33 per cent is reported. Microscopic examination reveals the presence of rosette aggregate crystals of calcium oxalate throughout the parenchyma. Most of the inorganic matter from the leaves seems to be extractable with water. Calcium, potassium and magnesium salts of organic acids are also present.

Cultivation Procedure

Soil

The crop thrives well on a variety of soils but is largely cultivated in sandy loam, red loam having even coarse gravelly soils, alluvial loam and rich clayey rice fields. Senna is also cultivated successfully in black cotton soils. When it is grown in high saline soils, plant growth is reduced without showing any excess injury symptoms. It can be successfully grown in soils ranging 7–8.5 pH. It is very sensitive to water-logging and, hence, it is grown only on well drained soil.

Climatic Requirements

Senna is a sun-loving crop and requires bright sunshine for its successful growth. It is usually cultivated as rainfed dry crop and very rarely as irrigated crop in certain areas. It is a deep rooted hardy plant and demands all around warm and dry weather conditions. The plant requires bright sun shine and occasional rains during its growth period. It is highly sensitive to heavy rainfall and water logging conditions. An average rainfall of 25–40 cm distributed from June to October is sufficient to yield good harvest. In south Indian condition, the crop may be grown as an early summer (Feb–March) or a winter (Oct–Nov)

Method of Propagation

Senna is generally propagated from seeds. Since the seed has a hard and tough covering, a certain amount of abrasion of its surface is helpful to induce quick germination. This may be done by grinding the seeds lightly with coarse sand in a morter (scarification)

Soaking the seeds for 10–12 hours before sowing is very much helpful to ensure germination.

About 15 kg of seeds are required for an hectare area of land in irrigated and 25–27 kg under rainfed condition. Bold, disease-free and mature seeds should be used for sowing.

The seed rate can be much lowered if the crop is grown as line sowing under irrigated condition. About 6 kg of seeds per hectare is found to be sufficient for optimum plant stand when the seeds are sown by dibbling.

The seeds are broadcast at a distance of 30 cm in lines made at 30 cm apart at 1.5–2.5 cm depth on well-prepared land. The germination starts on the third day and is completed within a fortnight. Before sowing, the field should be perfectly leveled, failing which, it hampers uniform germination. One light irrigation immediately after sowing improves germination.

The time of sowing seeds varies as per the onset of monsoon. In western India, June–July is optimum time of sowing. Seeds are sown soon after receiving first monsoon. Delay in sowing time considerably reduces vegetative growth phase at areas where winter sets by the end of October and as a result subsequent foliage yield is drastically reduced. However, in south India, the crop is sown in September–October, where it is grown under residual moisture after harvesting of paddy.

Land Preparation

The land is prepared deep and exposed to the sun for 110–115 days to dry out the roots of perennial weeds, followed by two cross-ploughing, harrowing and levelling. About 10 tonnes of FYM should be applied per hectare at the time of the final crossphoughing. The land is laid out into plots of convenient sizes making provision of irrigation channels.

Planting

Senna is generally directly shown in the field. But if the transplantation method is followed, transplanting is done when the seedlings are 10–15 days old. However, this method is less popular and not recommended for commercial cultivation.

Manuring

In most cases, the crop is grown economically by utilizing residual nutrients of previous crop and additional application of nutrients is usually not required. The farmers in south India use 5–10 tonns/ha of well-rotten FYM at the time of land preparation.

In international market, premium price is given for senna leaves grown organically. So ample use of manures is recommended for the crop grown for international market.

Irrigation

Senna is grown usually as a rainfed crop and in some areas, it is also grown under residual moisture. Therefore, in majority of growing areas no irrigation is provided except during prolonged drought. However, when the crop is grown as semi-irrigated crop, the yield increases considerably. In all, about 5–8 light irrigations are recommended to raise a good crop of senna. Two irrigations are however, very critical, the one immediately after sowing and the other at 30 days after. Heavy irrigation should be avoided as it is injurious to the crop.

Intercultural Measures

Three interculture operations are considered sufficient for the crop. The first one should be done 25–30 days after sowing, the next after 75–80 days and the third after 110–115 days. The growth of the crop is very slow at initial stage and requires care. Once the plant attains 20–25 cm height, they generally suppress weed growth.

Intercropping

Senna fits, well in crop rotation as khariff crop in commercially grown area. In south India, it is grown after the paddy and between rows of cotton, sesamum, chillies, brinjal, okra and tomatoes. In north India and western India, it is cropped only with mustard and coriander.

Crop Protection Measures

(1) *Damping-off Disease*

Seedlings are affected by the fungal species, *Rhizoctonia bataticola* rapidly if the seed beds and fields are affected by stagnating moisture at this stages and hence, drainage should be ensured.

(2) *Leaf-spot Disease*

This is the most serious disease and causes severe damage to the crop. The young and mature plants are infested and showed a severe leaf drop off resulting poor yield. The disease is caused by the fungi, *Alternaria alternate* (Fr.) Keisel and *Cerospora* species. Cloudy day and humid weather conditions are conducive for spread of the disease. The disease first appears on the leaves as visible minute spots and later turn dark brown to blackish patches. In case of serious infection, leaves start drying and falling. Pods are also affected in advanced stage of disease development.

(3) *Leaf-blight Disease*

Fully mature plants are affected in September–October in cloudy days and humid weather conditions by *Phyllosticta* fungi. This disease initially appears as small, brown, irregularly scattered lesions on leaves which grow bigger in size and turn black in colour at a later stage.

(4) *Leaf-eating Caterpillar of White Butterfly Attack*

Severe damage of foliage has been observed due to the caterpillar of *Catopsilia pyranthe.* The white butterfly lays eggs on the leaves of the crop and after hatching, the caterpillars feed on the leaves and remain active from July to October.

(5) *Pod-borer Attack*

Pod-borer is reported to attack the pods of mature plants and in storage conditions.

Harvesting

It has been found that, young senna leaves and pods contain a high sennoside content but since the produce is sold on the basis of weight, a balance between weight and content has to be made, to choose the right stage for harvest. It is also found that senna plants produce foliage containing higher sennosoids between 50–90 days of sowing.

The first picking of the foliage crop should be done at 50–70 days age when the leaves are fully grown, thick and bluish in colour, depending upon the total plant growth.

The picking of leaves is done by hand so that most of the growing tops are removed at harvest, this also induces more branching which, otherwise, reduces the foliage growth considerably.

A second picking is done at 90–100 days and the third picking between 140 –160 days when the entire plants are removed, for the leaves and pods collection togetherly.

For seed production, pods are collected during the month of February–March when the colour of the pods turns brown. Seeds from such harvest have high germination percentage.

Post-harvest Processing

The harvested crop should be spread in thin layer in an open field to reduce its moisture. Further drying of the produce is done in well-ventilated drying sheds. It takes 10–12 days to dry completely. Light green to greenish-yellow coloured dry leaves and pods are preferable in market. Improper and delayed drying changes the colour to black or brown which lowers the sennoside content and it fetches a lower price.

The pods are threshed during drying by beating pods with sticks to remove seeds.

Large leaves and bold pods with yellowish green in colour are in demand which fetch maximum price. Next grade of the produce is leaves and pods having brownish colour. Lowest grade of leaves in commerce is small and broken one.

On drying, the leaves are to be stored in cool and dry place. Pressing is done using hydraulic press to reduce the volume for transportation. The loss of sennioside contents in the stored produce is very slow and even after a year of storage, loss is negligible.

Yield

The yield of senna leaves may reach upto 15 q/ha (dry leaves) and 7q/ha of pods under irrigated and good management conditions. The yield under rainfed conditions is about 10q/ha of dry leaves and 4q/ha of pods.

Medicinal Properties

Senna is highly useful in chronic costiveness and in increasing peristaltic movements of colon. However, gripe by administering senna is also known especially when leaves are used. Regular use of senna is not desirable as it may even cause paralysis of intestine.

4.16 Long Pepper (Syn. Indian Long Papper)

Botanical Name

Piper longum Linn.

Indian Names

Hindi–Pipal, Pipli, Piplamul (root); *Bengali*–Piplamul (root); *Marathi*–Pimpli; *Gujarati*–Pipli; *Telugu*–Pippuloo; *Tamil*–Tippili; Pippili, Sirumulam, Kandan Tippili (root); *Kannada*–Hippali, Tippali; *Malayali*–Tippali, Pippali, Magadhi; *Sanskrit*–Magadhi, Pippali.

Botanical Family

Piperaceae.

Suitable Places for Growing in India

Commercial cultivation of the crop is distributed in West Bengal, Assam, Meghalaya, Maharastra (Akola region), Orissa, Andhra Pradesh (Vishakhapatnam), Uttar Pradesh, Tamil Nadu (Anaimalai Hills) and Kerala.

Botanical Description

Plant

A disecious perennial creeper, slender undershrub, root stock is erect, thick jointed and branched.

Stem

Stem numerous, glabrous, 0.6–0.9 m. long, ascending or prostrate (not climbing) much branched, stout, cylindrical, thickened above nodes, finely pubescent.

Leaves

Leaves simple, alternate, numerous, 6.3–9 cm long, lower ones broadly ovate, very cordate with all subacute, entire, glabrous, thin, buttate with reticulate venation sunk above and raised beneath, dark green and shining above, pale and dull beneath; petiole of lower leaves 5–7.5 cm, stout, of upper leaves very short or absent; stipules about 1.3 cm, membranous, lanceolate, obtuse, soon falling.

Flowers

Flowers are in solitary spikes, cylindrical, short and stout, peltate and adnate to the rachis, pendulate, male slender, bracts narrow; female 1.3–2.5 cm, bracts circular, flat, peltate; bracteoles when present forming low ridges on each side of the flower or connate in a semilunar form.

Perianth

Absent.

Androecium

Stamens 2; hypogynous; filament short; anther 2-celled; the cells distinct; dehiscent longitudinally.

Gynoecium

Ovary 1-celled; ovule solitary, terminal, erect; style short, conic, beaked; stigmas 3 or 4, short, spreading, persistent.

Fruit

Fruit very small, ovoid, completely sunk in solid, fleshy, berry over the spike, which is 2.5–3.8 cm, ovoid-oblong, erect, blunt, blackish green, shinning.

Seed

Seeds usually globose; testa thin; albumen floury within, with hardened periphery; embryo enclosed in an amniotic cavity at the end of the albumen remote from the hilum; cotyledons minute or obsolete; radical superior.

Species and Varieties

Based on the variations in the morphological character, it is being classified as Gol Tippili (West Bengal), Monsori (Maharastra), Asali and Suvali (Assam) and Soomai Tippali (Karnataka) An improved variety 'Viswa' was released by the Kerala Agricultural University.

Plant Parts Used

Thicker part of root and stem, spikes.

Chemical Component

Spike of *Piper longum*. Linn. has shown the presence of the alkaloids piperine (4–5 per cent) and piplartine and two new liquid alkaloids, one of which is designated as alkaloid A. Sesamin, dihydrostigmasterol and a new sterol, piplasterol are also present.

A sample of dried fruit of *P. longum* on steam distillation gave 0.7 per cent of an essential oil with spicy odour resembling that of pepper and ginger oils. The oil contained *n*-hexadecane (0.7 per cent); *n*-heptadecane (6.0 per cent); *n*-octadecane (5.3 per cent); *n*-nonadecane (5.8 per cent); *n*-eicosane (4.7 per cent); *n*-heneicosane (2.5 per cent); α-thujene (1.7 per cent); terpinolene (1.3 per cent); zingiberene, (7.0 per cent); *p*-cymene (1.3 per cent); *p*-methoxy acetophenone in trace amount; dihydrocarveol (4.3 per cent); phenethyl alcohol (2.1 per cent); and 2 new monocyclic sesquiterpenes (15.5 per cent, 11.1 per cent) respectively.

There are three grades of *Piplamul*, Grade I with thick roots and underground stems fetching higher price than Grade II or III, which comprise either thin roots, stems or broken fragments. Commercial drug consists almost entirely of transversely cut pieces (length, 5–25 mm; diam., 2–7 mm), which are cylindrical, straight or slightly curved, and some with distinct, swollen internodes showing a number of leaf and rootlet scars. The surface of the pieces is dirty, light brown in colour. The drug has a peculiar odour and a pungent bitter taste producing numbness on the tongue. It contains piperine (0.15–0.18 per cent), piplartine (0.13–0.20 per cent), and traces of a yellow crystalline pungent alkaloid. Other constituents found in the drug include triacontane, dihydrostigmasterol, an unidentified steroid, reducing sugars and glycosides. Two new alkaloids, named piperlongumine and piperlonguminine besides piperine have been isolated from the roots in another investigation.

Cultivation Procedure

Soil

The plant flourishes well in rich, well-drained and loamy soil. However it is also cultivated on a large scale in limestone soil at the Chirrapunji region. Laterite soils rich in organic matter with good moisture holding capacity are also considered and suitable. The plant can also be grown in well-drained fertile, black cotton soil.

Climatic Requirements

Long pepper is cultivated as a rainfed crop in Assam and Meghalaya region although grown as an irrigated crop in other parts where it is cultivated. The plant requires a hot moist climate and an elevation between 100 and 1000 m is suitable for its cultivation. It can be grown successfully even in areas which receive heavy rainfall with high relative humidity. In its natural habitat, the plant is found growing as an under shrub. The plant also requires partial shade (25 per cent) for its good growth.

Method of Propagation

Long pepper can be propagated through seeds, suckers or cuttings or by layering of mature branches at the beginning of rainy season. However, it can be easily propagated through the invigoration terminal stem cuttings obtained from one year old growth with 3 ? 5 internodes. Vine cuttings can be rooted in polythene bags filled with the common pot mixture. The nursery can be raised during March and April. The cuttings planted in March-April will be ready for planting in the field by the end of May. The rooting efficiency can be increased by treating the cuttings with bio-fertilizer slurry. The cuttings should be dipped in the slurry prepared by mixing 5g of *Azospirillum* sp. and 3 g of phosphobacteria in 100 ml water.

Land Preparation

Before planting, the land should be ploughed 2 to 3 times and leveled properly. The field is then divided into convenient size of plots in which pits are dug with a spacing of 60 cm × 60 cm. These pits should be filled with soil mixed with well-decomposed FYM or compost. In heavy rainfall areas, channels are necessary to be made to drain out excess water.

Planting

With the onset of monsoon, the rooted cuttings are planted in the pits at the rate of 2 per pit. The pits are gap filled one month after planting.

Transplanting of long pepper is done with the onset of monsoon in the month of May–June in West Bengal and in Kerala. In Maharashtra, planting is done in February end to middle of March.

Planting in done in such a way that atleast three to four nodes are buried in the soil and two nodes kept above the soil line. Sprouting starts usually within 15–20 days of planting.

Manuring

Tippili responds very well to organic manure. For the commercial cultivation, 20 tonns of FYM should be applied as basal dressing. During 2nd and 3rd year, FYM is spread in the root zone and mixed well with soil.

Irrigation

The crop should be irrigated once in a week in summer if it is grown as a pure crop. If grown as an intercrop, the irrigation that is provided to the main crop is sufficient. Sprinkler system of irrigation may be adopted for economising the irrigation water.

Intercultural Measures

Tippili requires staking for its proper growth. The stakes should be infixed within 3rd month of planting.

During the first year of planting, weeding becomes necessary. After the application of FYM to the beds, earthing should be done.

Mulching with organic mulches gives encouraging result especially when done in summer.

Intercropping

Long pepper is planted as an intercrop in subabul, eucalyptus, coconut, arecanut in different parts of the country.

Crop Protection Measures

Long pepper plants may be affected by the following insect pest and diseases –

(1) Mealy Bug Attack

During May–June, *Helopeltis theiveora* attacks the vegetative parts and spikes.

(2) ***Tea mosquito Bug Attack***

During May–June, young shoots and spikes are affected.

(3) ***Root and Leaf Rot Disease***

During rainy season *Colletotrichum* fungus attacks the plant and in summer season, *Colletotrichum* along with *Cercospora* species attack the plantation vigorously.

(4) ***Phytopthora Leaf and Stem Rot Disease:***

During rainy season, *Phytophthora* fungi attack the leaf and root.

Harvesting

The first harvest is done after six months of planting. The spikes become ready for harvest usually 2 months after their formation on the plants. Picking should be done when they are blackish green and most pungent.

In Kerala, three to four pickings are made depending upon the maturity of fruits.

Harvesting of over-mature or ripened fruits reduce the quality of the produce and makes difficulty to break easily after harvest.

After third year, the vines become less productive and hence, should be replanted.

Besides the spikes, the thick parts of the stems and roots which have medicinal value may also be harvested from 18 months after planting. At the time of harvesting, the stems are cut close to the ground and the roots are also dug up.

Post-harvest Processing

Spike

The harvested spikes are dried up in the sun for 4 to 5 days until they are thoroughly dried. The ratio of green to dry spike should be around 10 : 1.5. The dried spikes are stored in moisture-proof containers. The produce should not be stored for more than a year.

Stem and Root

Harvested stems and roots are cleaned and heaped in shade for a day, after which they are cut into 2.5 ? 5 cm long pieces. They are then graded and packed in gunny bags.

Yield

Spike

During the first year, the yield of dry spikes is about 400 kg/ha. The yield increases thereafter upto 3 years and the yield will be about 1000 kg/ha during the third year.

Root and Stem

The average yield of dried root and stem is about 500 kg/ha.

Medicinal Properties

The root is pungent, stomachic, laxative, anthelmintic, carminative, improves appetite, useful in bronchitis, abdominal pains, diseases of the spleen, tumours, biliousness etc.

The unripe fruit is somewhat sweetish, cooling and useful in biliousness.

The ripe fruit is pungent, sweetish, stomachic, aphrodisciac, alterative, laxative, antidiarrhoeic, antidysenteric and useful in abdominal complaints, fevers, leucoderma, urinary infection, tumours, piles, diseases of the spleen, leprosy, insomnia, jaundice, hiccough, tuberculous glands, biliousness and other diseases.

The fruit has a bitter and sharp taste. It is carminative, stomachic, emmenagogue, abortifacient, aphrodisciac, haematinic, diuretic, digestive and useful in inflammation of the liver, pains in the joints, lumbago, snake bite, scorpion-sting, night blindness.

In Travancore, an infusion of the root is prescribed after parturition, which facilitates in expulsion of the placenta.

In the Konkan region, the roasted spikes are beaten up with honey and given in rheumatism. They are also powered and mixed with black pepper, rock salt etc. (Two parts of long pepper, three of black salt and one part of salt)

4.17 Malabarnut (Syn. Vasaka)

Botanical Name

Adhatoda vasica Nees.

Indian Names

Bengali–Basak; *Gujarati*–Aradusi; *Hindi*–Arusa, Bansa; *Kannada*–Adusoga, Kurchigida, Pavate; *Malayali*–Adalodakam;

Orissi–Arusa, Basung; *Sanskrit*–Shwetavasa, Vasa, Vasaka; *Tamil*–Adhatodai, Pavettai; *Telugu*–Addasoramu, *Punjabi*–Bansa, Basuti, Bhekar, Vasaka.

Botanical Family

Acanthaceae.

Suitable Places for Growing in India

The shrubs can be grown in tropical and sub-tropical regions India.

Botanical Description

Plant

A dense shrub of 1.2–2.4 m height with many long ascending branches.

Stem

Stem stout with yellowish bark, terete, glabrous.

Leaves

Length 12.5– 20 and width 3.8–6.3 cm; elliptic-lanceolate, acuminate, minutely puberulose when young, glabrous when mature, entire, dark green above, paler beneath, base tapering; main nerves 10–12 pairs with reticulate venation between; petioles 1.3–2.5 cm long.

Flowers

Flowers in short, dense, axillary pedunculate spikes of 2.5–7.5 cm length, towards the end of the branches; peduncles 3.8–10 cm, stout, shorter than the leaves; bracts reaching 2.2 by 1.3 cm, elliptic, subacute, glabrous or nearly so, 5– 7 nerved, closely reticulately veined; bracteoles 20 by 4 mm, oblong-lanceolate, acute, with ciliolate margins, 1-nerved, reticulately veined.

Calyx

Sepals less than 1.3 cm long, glabrous or slightly pubescent, divided within 2 mm of the base, segments imbricate, oblong–lanceolate, acute, 3-nerved, reticulately veined.

Corolla

Coralla white, with a few irregular rose-coloured bars in the throat, 3.2 cm long, pubescent outside, tube 1.3 cm long, the lower half cylindric, 4 mm diam., the upper half much laterally inflated; upper lip 2 by 1.3 cm long, ovate-oblong, curved, obtuse, notched, lower lip as long as the upper, the lobes 1.3 cm deep, oblong, rounded, the middle lobe the broadest.

Androecium

Stamens 2, inserted near the top of the coralla tube, filaments hairy at the very base, long, stout, curved; anthers 2-celled, lower anther-cells minutely apiculate (not white-spurred) at the base.

Gynoecium

Ovary pubescent, 2-celled, ovules 2 in each cell; lower part of the style pubescent, filiform, subclavate above; stigma entire.

Fruit

Capsules 1.9–2.2 by 0.8–0.9 cm, cleavate, subacute, shortly and bluntly pointed, pubescent, solid stalk flattened, 1 cm long.

Seeds

Seeds usually 1 or 2, 6 by 5 mm long, orbicular-oblong, tubercular-verrucose, glabrous.

Plant Parts Used

Leaves, bark.

Chemical Components

The following alkaloids are present in different parts of the plants.

Vasicine	(Leaves, inflorescence, flowers, stems and roots),
l-*Vasicinone*	(Leaves),
Vasicinol	(Leaves and roots)
Vasicinine	(Inflorescence, flowers, stems and roots),
Vasicoline	(Whole young plant),
Vasicolinone	(Whole young plant),
Adhatodine	(Whole young plant),
Anisotine	(Whole young plant),

The alcoholic extract of the dried leaves shows atropine like activity due to the presence of a non-nitrogenous and non-toxic principle, vasakin. It is a white, non-crystalline steroid. It is soluble in petroleum ether. Vasakin exhibits hypoglycaemic activity, but is less potent than tolbutamide.

The leaves contain betaine, an essential oil, fats, resins, sugar, mucilage, adhatodic acid, a yellow dye, tritriacontane (0.075 per cent) and β-sitosterol (0.013 per cent) The leaves are rich in vitamin C (up to 250 mg/100 g) and carotene (4,500 μg/100 g) On steam distillation, the leaves yield a fragrant, golden yellow, essential oil (0.075 per cent on dry basis); it is also present in the roots and flowers. The oil contains limonene. The physico-chemical properties and constituents of the essential oil are not yet fully known.

The petroleum ether extract of the leaves yields a resin. It has expectorant action, but is less potent than the essential oil. The resin, on stem–and vacuum-distillation, yields limonene and oxygenated bodies of high boiling points. The resin which is cheaply and easily available, is reported to be toxic grain insects, though less so than Malathion; it is non-toxic to man. Besides the resin, the extract also contains hentriacontane and phytosterol.

Flower showed the presence of vasicine (inflorescences 0.64 per cent; flowers 0.15 per cent on dry basis) and vasicinine (inflorescences 0.68 per cent; flowers 0.35 per cent on dry basis) The inflorescences also contained β-sitosterol (up to 0. 035 per cent) The flowers yield a golden yellow essential oil. The colouring matter in the flowers includes luteolin, quercetin and kaempferol. Other non-nitrogenous constituents include α-amyrin, tritriacontane (flowers, 0.07 per cent; flowering tops 0.09 per cent on dry basis), and β-sitosterol.

The root is administered as a decoction along with other expectorants. It contains vasicine and vasicinol and tritriacontane (0.0.7 per cent) The roots also contain an essential oil.

The seeds on extraction with petroleum ether produce a deep yellow, fatty oil (25.8 per cent) The fatty acid composition of the oil is as follows: arachidic (3.1 per cent); behenic (11.2 per cent); lingnoceric (10.7 per cent); cerotic (5.0 per cent); oleic (49.9 per cent); and linoleic (12.3 per cent) The absence of stearic and palmitic acids and the presence of the cerotic acid are unusual features of the oil. β-Sitosterol has been isolated from the unsaponifiable matter.

Cultivation Procedure

Soil

It flourishes well in rich, well-drained loamy soil. However, it is also cultivated on a large scale in limestone soil at the Chirrapunji region. Laterite soils rich in organic matter with good moisture holding capacity are also considered suitable. It can also be grown in well-drained, fertile, black cotton soil.

Climatic Requirements

The plant requires a hot moist climate and an elevation between 100 and 1000 m. It can be easily grown even in areas which receives heavy rainfall with high relative humidity.

Method of Propagation

Vasaka can be easily propagated by seeds and stem cuttings. Terminal stem cuttings obtained from one year old growth of pencil thickness with 3–5 internodes show better rooting. Stem cuttings can be rooted in polythene bags filled with common pot mixture. For nursery propagation, nursery can be raised during March ? April. The cuttings may be planted in May–June and will be ready for field plantation by the end of July.

Land Preparation

Before planting, the land should be ploughed 2–3 times and leveled properly at least one month before. Then the field is divided into convenient size of plots in which pits are dug at least one month before planting at a spacing of 2 m × 3 m and the pits should be 50 cm × 50 cm × 5 cm in size. These pits should be filled with soil mixed with well-decomposed FYM or compost. In heavy rainfall areas, channels are made to drain out excess water.

Planting

The rooted cuttings are planted in the pits at the rate of 2 per pit by the end of July. The pits are gap-filled again one month after planting.

Manuring

Vasaka responds well to organic manure. For commercial cultivation, 20 tonns of FYM are applied as basal dressing. During next several years, same amount of FYM is spread near the root zone and mixed well with soil.

Irrigation

The crop should be irrigated once in a week if it is grown as a pure crop at least after six months after plantation. In case, the crop is grown as an intercrop with other crops, the irrigation provided to the main crop is sufficient. Sprinkler system of irrigation may be adopted for economising the irrigation water. After six months of plantation when the crop become healthy, irrigation may be done fortnightly when the soil becomes dry.

Intercultural Measures

During the first year of the planting, weeding and hoeing are done when weed growth is found in the field. After the application of FYM to the pits, earthing-up is done from the channels. Pruning may be done before rainy season for better vegetative growth.

Intercropping

Vasaka may be planted as an intercrop in coconut, arecanut, ginger plantations etc.

Crop Protection Measures

Vasaka plants may be affected by the following diseases.

(1) Greasy Rust Disease

During the monsoon season, *Chnoopsora butleri* Diet and Syd. attack the young and mature plants.

(2) Other Fungal Disease

During summer and rainy season the following fungi may attack the plantation –

(a) *Nectria flavoviridis* Wollenw.
(b) *Alternaria alternata* (Fr.) Keissler.
(c) *Chaetomium globosum* Kunze. & Schm.
(d) *Colletotrichum capsici* (Syd) Butler & Bisby.
(e) *Botryodiplodia theobromae* Pat.
(f) *Nigrospora oryzae* (Berk. & Br.) Petch.
(g) *Drechslera speciferum* (Bain.) Nicot.
(h) *Phyllosticta vasicae* Pandotra & Ganguly.

Harvesting

The first harvest from the field may be done after 6 years of planting. Before the onset of monsoon, the leaves and during winter season the bark are generally collected.

Post-harvest Processing

Leaves

The harvested leaves are dried in shade and stored in gunny bags.

Bark

Bark is collected by scalping the stems and trunk. Harvested barks are cut into pieces and dried and stored in moisture proof container.

Yield

Under irrigated conditions, about 1–1.5 tonnes/ha of leaves may be obtained from the field.

The average yield of dried bark is 200–250 kg/ha in every year after six years of plantation.

Medicinal Properties

The plant parts are pungent, bitter, acrid, cooling, useful in bronchitis, leprosy, blood impurities, heart troubles, thirst, asthma, fever, vomitting, loss of memory, leucoderma, consumption, jaundice, tumours, diseases of the mouth etc. The root facilitates the expulsion of the foetus, useful in strangury, and in leucorrhoea with blood discharges.

The root is diuretic, useful in bronchitis, asthma, bilious vomitting, sore eyes, fevers, gonorrhoea. The leaves are emmenagogue and useful in gonorrhoea. The flowers improve the circulation of the blood, lessen strangury and jaundice. The fruit is useful in bronchitis.

The leaves and the roots of this plant are considered very efficacious remedy for all sorts of coughs, cold and administered with ginger. The leaves are also used for rheumatism.

In West Bengal leaves are dried and made into cigarettes and smoked in asthma and their juice is used for diarrhoea and dysentery.

The flowers, leaves, roots and especially the flowers are supposed to possess antispasmodic qualities. They are bitterish and sub-aromatic and are administered in infusion and electuary as antihelminthic.

The flowers and the fruits are bitter, aromatic and antispasmodic. The fresh flowers are used in ophthalmia.

The Burmese pound the leaves and use them as a poultice for fresh wounds, while an infusion of the leaves and twigs is given internally for coughs. In the Tenasserim district, the leaves are used externally in case of swellings, bleeding of the nose and headache and internally for fever, colic, asthma and dysentery. It has been known to cure bleeding of the lungs by taking a sweetened decoction of the plant and the preparation is an excellent mixture for children and others for cough and colds.

In Sri Lanka, the whole plant is used in the treatment of excessive phlegm and also in menorrhagia.

The plant especially the leaf is credited with antiseptic and parasiticidal properties.

4.18 Periwinkle (Syn. Madagascar or Red or White Periwinkle, Old Maid)

Botanical Name

***Catharanthus roseus* (L.) G. Don.**

Indian Names

Bengali–Gulferinghi, Nayantara; *Gujarati*–Baramasi; *Hindi*–Sadabahar, Sada Suhagan, Madan, Mainphal; *Kannada*–Kanpukasi Kanegale, Kasikanagile Smashna Mallige, Smashana Kanagale; *Tamil*–Madkarai, Marukkalankay, Sudukadumallikai; *Telugu*–Billaganneru; *Malayali*–Ushamalari; *Marathi*–Sadaphul; *Orissi*–Ainskuti; *Punjabi*–Rattanjot.

Botanical Family

Apocynaceae.

Suitable Places for Growing in India

It is naturally grown as wild and mostly naturalized upto an altitude of 1,3000 m and commonly grown in gardens throughout the country.

It is cultivated in Tamil Nadu, Karnataka, Andhra Pradesh, Madhya Pradesh, Gujarat and Assam.

Botanical Description

Plant

It is a perennial herb, erect, branched, and is about 1 m height.

Stem

Stem is erect, lax branching with flexible long branches and laticiferous tissues prevails in its aerial parts.

Leaves

Leaf simple, opposite, ex-stipulate, petiolate, oblong-obovate, acute, rounded apex, smooth with entire margin, upper laminary surface deeper green and glossy than lower surface where the veins are prominent, slightly foetid, 4–10 cm by 2–4 cm.

Flower

Flowers in axilary or terminal cymes, solitary or paired or clustered. Flowers are rose-purple or white or white with a rose-purple or yellow spot in the centers or orifice region, shortly pedicillate, harmaphrodite, complete, actinomorphic and hypogynous.

Calyx

Sepals 5, calyx lobes are linear, subulate.

Corolla

Petals 5, corolla tube is cylindrical, measures upto 30 cm in length, rose-purple or white or white with a rose-purple spot in the center, tubular, swollen in the region of the epipetalous anthers, the throat of the corolla-tube is hairy, forming a corona-like structure.

Androceium

Stamens 5, included in the corolla tube, filaments are very small, epipetalous, anthers are borne inside the bulging distal end of corolla tube convering conically above the stigma and anthers sagittarious.

Gynoecium

Ovaries 2, free below but united in the stylar region; carpels-2, stigma 1, dumbel-shaped, which is ascribed to post-genital carpel fusion. After fertilization, the carpels separate and from two fruits.

Fruits

Fruit mericarp, dehiscent with a pair of hairy follicles each measuring about 22–25 mm in length and 2.3–3 mm in diametre and contain upto 30 linearly arranged seeds.

Seed

Seeds are small, black in colour, covered with a thin black tegument. On maturity, the follicles split along the length dehiscing the seeds and 1 g contains about 835–838 seeds.

Species and Varieties

There are 3 varieties in piriwinkle, those with (*i*) Rose-pruple flowers, (*ii*) white flowers and (*iii*) white flowers with a rose-purple or yellow spot in the centre.

Rose-purple flowers are described as cultivar "Rosea", white flowers are "Alba" and the third one is "Ocellata".

The first type is being cultivated because of its higher alkaloid content. Recently two white-flowered varieties named "Nirmal" and "Dhawal" have been released by the CIMAP, Lucknow.

Plant Parts Used

Stem, foliage, root.

Chemical Component

The following alkaloids are present in various parts of the plants.

Ajmalicine (raubasine, δ-yohimbine, vinceine, vincaine, tetrahydroserpentine), 14, 15-Dehydroepivincadine, Akuammicine, N-Demethylvinblastine, Akummine, (vincamajoridine), Deoxyvinblastine (isoleurosine), Alstonine, 4-Desacetoxy-hydroxyvinblastine, Ammocalline, Dihydrositsirikine, Ammorosine, Fluorocarpamine, Amotin, Fluorocarpamine-N-oxide, Bannucine, Gomaline, β-Carboline, (norharmane), 19-Hydroxytabersonine, Carosidine, Isositsirikine, Carosine, Z-Isositsirikine, Catharanthamine, Leurocolombine, Catharanthine, Leurosidine (vinleurosidine, vinrosidine), Catharicine, Leurosidine-N'b-oxide, Catharine, Leurosine (vinleurosine), Cathindine, Leurosine, Cathovaline, Leurosinone, Cavincidine, Leurosivine, Cavincine, Lochnericine, Coronaridine, Lochneridine, Deacetoxyvinblastine,

Lochnerine, Deacetylvincaleukoblastine, Lochnerinine, Deacetylvindoline, Lochnerivine, Deacetylvindorosine, (catharosine), Lochrovicine, N-Deformylvincristine, Lochrovidine, Lochrovine, Vinamidine (catharinine), Maandrosine, Vinaphamine, 11-Methoxytabersonine, Vinaspine, Mitraphylline, Vinblastine (vincaleukoblastine), Neoleurocristine, Vincadioline, Neolcurosidine, Vincaline, Pericathidine, Pericyclivine, Vincamicine, Perimivine, Vincarodine, Perividine, Vincathicine, Perivine, Vincolidine, Perosine, Vincoline, Pleiocarpamine, Vincoside, Pleurosine (leurosine-N'b-oxide), Vincristine (leurocristine, vincaleurocristine), Pseudovinblastinediol, Vincubine, Reserpine, Vindolicine, Rhazimol, Vindolidine, Rosamine, Vindoline, Roseadine, Vindolinine, Roseamine, Vindolinine-N-oxide, Rosicine, 19S-Vindolinine, Rovidine, 19S-Vindolinine-N-oxide, Rozevin, Serpentine, Vinosidine, Sitsirikine, Vinsedicine, Tabersonine, Vinsedine, Tetrahydro-alstonine, Virosine, Venalstonine.

Cultivation Procedures

Soil

The crop is quite hardy and grows well on a wide variety of soils, except those which are alkaline or water-logged. Deep sandy loam to loamy soils of medium fertility with a pH of upto 8.5 are preferred for its large-scale cultivation, as in this soil there is not only a better development of roots, but is also easy to pull them out for harvest.

Climatic Requirement

The distribution of the plant makes it apparent that there is no specificity in its climatic requirements. It comes up well in tropical and subtropical areas. However, the growth in tropical areas is better than in the subtropical areas, where its growth is slow due to low temperature in winter. The crop prefers warm, dry conditions all round the year and remains for 200 days in field. Where rainfall is high and well-distributed, it can be grown as a rainfed crop. It can be successfully grown up to an elevation of 1,300 m above sea-level.

Method of Propagation

Perwinkle can be propagated from seeds or soft-wood cuttings. Since plants propagated by cuttings flower earlier than those from seed-propagated plant, it is recommended that for drug production, the plants should be grown from seeds and for seed production, plants are to be raised form cuttings.

Fresh seeds collected a few months in advance are preferred for sowing, as they lose viability on storage. The seeds can either be directly sown in the field or in a nursery bed and the seedlings are transplanted.

In direct sowing, the seeds at the rate of 2.5 kg/ha are broadcast at the onset of the monsoon in June-July, in lines 30–45 cm apart and then lightly covered with fine leaf-mould. Since the seeds are very small, for better handling and distribution, they are mixed with sand and leaf-mould mixture in 1: 1 ratio, about 10 times of their weight. In directly sown fields, a light irrigation needs to be given, if it does not rain in next 2 days. Seeds germinate within 7–8 days. After 30–45 days of germination, the seedlings are thinned at a spacing of 30 cm within the row.

In nursery transplanting method, the seeds are sown in well-prepared, raised nursery beds in March-April by broadcasting them in rows spaced at 8–10 cm apart and at about 1.5 cm depth. They are then covered with a light soil and leaf-mould mixture at 1: 1 ratio and watered to keep the bed moist. For nursery, 500 g seed produce enough seedlings to plant an hectare area of land. Seeds germinate within 10 days of sowing.

In vegetative propagation, soft-wood cuttings obtained from the lateral soots are better than the semi-hard wood cuttings. Cuttings of more than 10–15 cm length with a minimum of 5–6 nodes are recommended for vegetative propagation. Soaking the cuttings overnight in 25–50 ppm of NAA solution shows 90 per cent rooting. The rooted cuttings are then ready for transplanting which is done at a spacing of 45 × 30 cm apart in the field.

Land Preparation

The land is repeatedly ploughed and brought to a fine tilth and weeds, stubbles, pebbles etc. are to be removed. The field is divided into plots of convenient size and the soil is mixed with recommended dose of manures. About 25 tonns of FYM is required for an hectare area of land. Groundnut cake, bone-meal, rapeseed-cake and vermicompost are also beneficial for better growth of the plants. To remove mites and nematods from the field, prior application of neem cake is recommended at the doses of 7–12 kg/ha.

Planting

The 60-day old seedlings, which are 12–15 cm tall, are ready for transplanting. The seedlings are transplanted at a spacing of 45 cm × 30 cm apart in the field. A plant population of 75,000 plants/ha is optimum.

Manuring

In low fertile soil, 20–25 tonns of FYM/ha is recommended but in moderately fertile condition the dose may be reduced at 15–18 tonns/ha. If irrigation facilities are available, it is recommended to green manure the field leguminous crops. The seeds of the green manure crop may be treated with the bacterial inoculants before sowing so as it increase the development of root nodules which absorb atmospheric nitrogen and fix it into the soil.

Irrigation

The plants are drought-resistant but light irrigation in hot-weather is much helpful. In comparison to stem and roots, leaves showed higher concentration of alkaloid under soil moisture deficit condition.

Intercultural Measures

The crop is given 2–3 intercultures at internal of 20 or 30 days. Once the plants cover the field, they smother weed growth. Mulching with rice straw or cut-grass is recommended to minimize weed growth.

At early flowering stage, the top 2 cm portions of the plant are removed to promote vegetative growth and alkaloid content.

Intercropping

The crop may be grown as an itnercrop in *Eucalyptus* or other plantations.

Crop Protection Measures

Periwinkle crop is sufficiently hardy and relatively free from the damages due to pests and diseases. However, in some areas, the crop faces some attack, which are as follows.

(1) ***Termites and Other Soil-borne Insects Attack***

They may be effectively controlled by application of neem-cake or other neem-based biopesticides before planting.

2) ***Thrips and Aphids Attack***

Decoction made from tobacco leaves and other plant materials are helpful to control these pests.

3) ***Green Rosettae Viral Disease***

Atrophy is noted at all the growing parts and at any stage of growth.

Affected plants should be removed.

(4) ***Cucumber Mosaic Viral Disease***

Several leaf mosaics occur at any stage of growth of the plants and affected plants should be removed.

(5) ***Little-leaf Disease***

In Orissa, the infestation caused by MLO-mycoplasma is found in young plants, the leaves and flowers become small and green fruit formation stops. The disease is transmitted through grafts.

(6) ***Damping-off Disease***

Seedlings stage of plant are attacked by this disease caused by *Phytophthora parasitica* Dastur, *Pythium butleri* Subram., *Fusarium* species.

(7) ***Leaf-spot Disease***

During July-August the young plants are affected by *Alternaria alternata* (Fr.), *Myrothesium yoridum*, *Alternaria tenuissima*, *Rhizoctonia solani*, *Ohiobolus catharanthicola*, *Haplosporella marathwadenis*, *Glomerella cingulata*.

(8) ***Die-back Disease***

Young plants are affected by this disease showing twig blight or top rot symptoms caused by *Pythium butleri*, *Phytophthora nicotianae*, *P. debaryanum* etc.

(9) ***Fungal Attack***

The young plants are affected during the monsoon season by the fungi, *viz.*, *Alternaria tenuissima* and *Colletotrichum dematium*.

(10) Fusarium Wilt Disease

The fungi responsible are *Fusarium solani, Sclerotium roffsii.*

(11) Blight Disease

Young plants are attacked by the fungus, *Pythium aphanidermatum.*

Harvesting

Roots

The crop is ready for harvest after 12 months of sowing. About 150 days after sowing or transplanting, the periwinkle roots penetrate the soil upto 15–20 cm and then produce lateral rootlets. The plants are cut about 7.5 cm above the ground level dried for the stems, leaves and the seeds. The field is then copiously irrigated and when the field reaches the proper condition for digging, it is ploughed and the roots are collected and washed.

Leaves, Stems and Seeds

Two leaf strippings are done, the first after 6 months and second after 9 months of sowing. Third leaf stripping is also obtained when whole plant is harvested.

The leaves and stems are collected separately. The aerial part of the plant between 7.5 cm and about 25 cm above the ground level is taken as the stem crop after whole plant is harvested.

In case of seeds, they are collected after the plant is harvested and dried in the shade. The seed pod dehisces and release the seeds with a light threshing.

Post-harvest Processing

Root

The roots are washed properly, then cut into pieces of 15–25 cm length and dried.

Stem

The basal stems upto about 10 cm long are separated from roots and cut into pieces and dried.

Leaves

The harvested leaves are dried in shade and stored.

Seeds

Seeds are collected by a light threshing to the dried seed pods of harvested dried plants.

Yield

Under irrigated conditions, about 4 tonnes/ha of leaves,1.5 tonnes/ha of roots and 1.5 tonnes/ha of stems on an dried basis may be obtained. Whereas, the yield under rainfed condition may be about 2 tonnes/ha of leaves and 0.75 tonnes/ha of stem and root on died basis.

Under south Indian condition, the total yield in respect of leaves, stems and roots comes to about 2.2 tonnes/ha from an irrigated crop and in the north Indian plains, the yield may go upto 1.8 tonnes/ha.

Medicinal Properties

Vinblastine, vincristine, leurosidine and leurosine are oncolytic alkaloids, that are present in all parts of the plants and are effective against P-1534 loukaemia. Vinbalstine sulphate, another alkaloid present in all parts of the plant, is used particularly to treat Hodgkin's disease besides lymphosarcoma, choriocarcinoma, neuroblastoma, carcinoma of the breast, lungs and other organs in acute and chronic leukaemia. It is also used against Wilms' Tumour, neuroblastoma, rhabdosarcoma and reticulum cell sarcoma.

Besides anti-leukaemic activity, the total alkaloids and chloroform extracted crude showed significant tranquilizing properties. The alkaloids also cause relaxant and antispasmodic effect on the smooth muscles of the intestine and uterus.

4.19 Rauvolfia (Syn. Serpentine or Serpentina Root)

Botanical Name

Rauvolfia serpentina **Benth. Ex. Kurz.**

Common Names

Sanskrit–Sarpagandha, Chundrika; Urd.–Asrel; Hind.–Chandrabhaga, Chota-chand; *Bengali*–Chandar; *Marathi*–Harkaya, Harki; *Telugu*–Paataala-gani, Paataala Garuda; *Tamil*–Chivan Amelpodi; *Kannada*–Sarpagandhi, Shivanabhiballi, Sutranavi, Patalagandhi; *Malayali*–Chuvannavilpori, Suvapaval-poriyan; *Orissi*–Patalgarur, Sanochado.

Botanical Family

Apocynaceae.

Suitable Places for Growing in India

It is commercially cultivated in Uttar Pradesh, Bihar, Orissa, West Bengal, Assam, Andhra Pradesh, Tamil Nadu, Kerala, Karnataka and Maharastra. It is naturally found widely in the Himalayan foothills and peninsular India.

Botanical Description

Plant

A small erect shrub rarely reaching 0.9 m high; bark pale, rarely lenticellate.

Stem

Stem stout, erect, softy woody.

Leaves

Leaves in whorls of 3, thin, 7.5–18 by 2.5–6.3 cm, lanceolate, acute or acuminate, glabrous, bright green above, pale beneath, base tapering; main nerves 8–10 pairs, slender, petioles 8 mm long, somewhat obscure owing to the blade running down into the petiole.

Flowers

Flowers white, often tinged with violet, in many flowered irregular corymbose cymes; peduncles 5–12.5 cm long; pedicles stout, 3–6 mm long, bright red; bracts beneath the pediclels triangular, acute, 1–1.5 mm long.

Calyx

Calyx short, 5-fid, glandular inside. Calyx glabrous, bright red; segments 2.5–3.0 mm long, lanceolate.

Corolla

Corolla–hypocrateriform; inflated over the anthers; usually hairy within; corolla 1–1.3 cm long; tube slender, swollen a little above the middle; lobes 5, 3 mm long, elliptic-oblong, rounded at the apex, overlapping to the left.

Androecium

Stamens 5, inserted at the middle of the corolla tube or higher up, included; filaments usually short; anther cells 2, anthers small, subacute, the cells rounded at the base, dehiscing longitudinally.

Gynoecium

Disks cup shaped, membranous, obscurely lobed carpels-2, distinct or connate; ovules 2 in each carpel, collateral; style filiform; stigma thick, broad and often toothed at the apex, annular or appendiculate at the base, tip shortly 2-fid.

Fruit

Drups single, or didymous and connate more or less deeply, about 6–6.2 mm diameter, purplish black when ripe.

Seed

Seed ovoid; albumen fleshy; colyledons flat.

Species and Varieties

Besides *Rouwolfia serpentina* Benth. Ex Hurz., another species *R. tetraphylla* also grown widely. RS-1 variety, released from Jawaharlal Nehru Krishi Vishswa Vidyalaya, College of Agriculture, Indore, contain high percentage of alkaloid at eighteen months of age.

Plant Parts Used

Root.

Chemical Component

The following alkaloids are present in the serpentine roots.

Canembine, Ajmalidine, Corynanthine, Ajmaline, Seredine, Mauiensine, Yohimbine, Isoajmaline, α-Yohimbine, Mitoridine β-Yohimbine, Picrinine, Purpeline, Rauvomitine, Rauwolfinine, Sandwicine, ψ-Yohimbine, Seredamine, Tetraphyllicine, Deserpidine, Vincamajine, Isopseudoreserpine, Vomalidine, Isoranecscine, Isoreserpine, Raugustine, Isoreserpiline-Ψ-indoxyl, Raunescine, Renoxidine, Perakine, Rescidine, Vomilenine, Rescinnamine, Reserpic acid methyl ester, Carapanaubine, Reserpine, Rauvoxine, ψ-Reserpine, Rauvoxinine, Deserpideine, Ajmalinine, Raujemedine, Alkaloid A, Alkaloid D, Ajmalicine, Alkaloid RP1, Aricine, Alkaloid RP2, Isoreserpiline, Alkaloid RP3, Isoreserpinine, Amsoniaefoline, Rauniticine, Raunitidine, Chandrine, Raumitorine, Neoreserpiline, Rauvanine, Obscuridine,

Reserpiline, Obscurine, Reserpinine, Pelirine, Tetrahydroalstonine, Raucaffricine, Tetraphylline, Raucaffridine, Raucaffriline, Alstonine, Raunamine, Serpentine, Rauwolfine, Serpentinine, Sandwicensine, Neosarpagine, Samatine, Sarpagine, Semperflorine.

Cultivation Procedure

Soil

The plant grows in a wide variety of soils, from sandy alluvial loam to red lateritic loam or stiff dark loam. In its natural habitat, it prefers clay or clayey loam with a large percentage of humus, and it does not grow well in soil having pH 8 or above. The ideal pH for this crop is from 4.6–6.2. The plant produces thicker roots in black, stiff loam soils than in heavy clayey or sandy soil. Soils containing large quantities of sand, retard the growth of the plants and make them move susceptible to root and leaf disease.

Climatic Requirements

This plant can be grown under a wide range of climatic conditions. It flourishes in hot, humid condition and can be grown both in the sun and in partial shade. It prefers tropical to sub-tropical climate, receiving heavy monsoon rains between June and August preferably the South-West.

In Deccan peninsula region, where more equitable climate remains throughout the year as compared to the sub-Himalayan tracts, are said to be more suitable for a commercial cultivation of this plant. A climate with a temperature range of 10–30°C are seems to be the best for this plant. In low rainfall areas, the plant can be successfully cultivated, if irrigation is available during the drier months. Though the plant seems to be sensitive to water-logging, it can withstand water for 2–3 days without too much damage. The plant sheds its leaves during the cold months in localities with severe winters. Frost kills the top tender, green twigs only and fresh shoots sprout up with the advent of spring from the thicker shoots which can withstand the frost.

Method of Propagation

R. serpentina can be propagated by seeds, root cutings, root stumps and stem cuttings.

Direct sowing of seeds in the field has not been found successful and hence seedling are raised in the nursery and transplanted in the field. The germination percentage of seeds is very poor and variable (25–50 per cent) This is attributed partly to the adverse influence of the stony endocarp. A more serious factor is that in many species of the genus in both the hemispheres, fruits of perfectly normal external appearance contain no embryos, an effect possibly of parthenocarpy or of deferred somatoplastic sterility.

Recently, it has been found that fresh seeds collected from ripe fruits, immediately before sowing showed a germination rate of 58–74 percent. A delay of 24–36 hours between collection and sowing of seeds reduced their rate of germination. Sun-dried and stored seeds generally gave a low rate of germination and seeds stored for more than 7–8 months practically did not germinate. The ripe seeds, collected from the beginning of June to the end of October or even November and stored in air-tight tins, retained their viability for about six months.

For propagation by root cuttings, large tap-roots with a few filiform lateral secondary rootlets are used. Cuttings, 2.5–5.0 cm long are planted horizontally about 5 cm below the surface or in holes. They are irrigated and nearly 50 percent of the root cuttings, planted at the beginning of the monsoon sprout in about a month. Trials at Dehra Dun and other places have shown that under irrigated conditions root cuttings of about 0.25 cm diameter planted during March–June gave 52–79 percent success. In another study, cuttings of 1.25 cm diameter rooted within 10–15 days, producing healthy roots and shoots. Thicker roots, split into pieces of 1.25 diameter, have also been found to produce shoots normally. About 100 kg of root cuttings are required to plant a hectare area of land. The high percentage of successful plants obtained by root cuttings makes it preferable to propagation by seeds. However, the alkaloidal content of roots from them has been found to be not so high as in plants raised from seeds.

Propagation by root stumps was attempted using about 5 cm of root with a portion of stem above the collar. This method met with about 90–95 percent success or sometimes even 100 percent. Such plants transplanted in May–July in irrigated fields, become well established by the end of September. This method, however, has its limitation in that only one plant can be raised from a single stump.

Stem cuttings taken from woody twigs have also been tried for propagation. Hardwood cuttings have been found better than softwood cuttings; cuttings, 15.0–23.0 cm long, having three internodes are most suitable. Highest percentage (60–100 per cent) of rooting was obtained by treating hardwood cuttings with β-indolyl acetic acid solution (30 ppm) for 12 hours; treated cuttings rooted within 15 days. Stem cuttings planted in the nursery during early monsoon (June), and kept moist until they sprout, have given 40–65 percent success. Such cuttings, though they start sprouting 3–4 days after planting, actually strike root mostly after about 75 days. Premonsoon planting has not been successful, in spite of copious irrigation and protection against sun. Stem cuttings have been found less satisfactory than root cuttings, since many of them do not root easily.

Land Preparation

The land is repeatedly ploughed and brought to a fine tilth and weeds, stubbles, pebbles are to be removed from the field. The field is divided into plots of convenient size and the soil is mixed with recommended dose of manures. About 20–25 tones of FYM is required for an hectare area of land. Groundnut cake, bone-meal, rapeseed-cake and vermicompost are also beneficial for better growth of the plants. To remove the mites and nematods from the field, prior application of neem cake is recommended at the doses of 7–12 kg/ha.

Planting

The rooted cuttings are transplanted in the field at a spacing of 45 cm × 30 cm apart in the field. A plant population of 75,000 plants/ha is optimum.

Manuring

In low fertile soil, 20–25 tonns of FYM/ha is recommended but in moderate fertile condition, the dose may be reduced at 15–18 tonns/ha. If irrigation facilities are available, it is recommended to green manure the field with leguminous crops. The seeds of the green manure crop may be treated with the bacterial inoculants prior to sowing to increase the development of root nodules which absorb atmospheric nitrogen and fix it in the soil.

Irrigation

The crop may be irrigated fortnightly in the hot dry season and about once a month in winter. The crop can be cultivated under rainfed conditions, but the yield is considerably poorer.

Intercultural Measures

In order to maintain the satisfactory development of roots about 2–3 weedings are necessary during the monsoon and one hoeing at the end of the growing season (December)

Intercropping

Soyabeans, onions and garlic may be grown as intercrop with the serpentiana, but the yield of serpentina roots was reported to be higher as monocrop system. It can also be grown as an intercrop with maize, cowpea, brinjal during kharif and radish, wheat or cole crop during rabi season.

Crop Protection Measures

R. serpentian plants may be affected by the following insect, pest and diseases.

(1) *Root Knot Disease*

Root knots appear as galls of various sizes, covering the root system. Stunted growth of plants, etiolation and decreases in leaf size are the symptom in the arial portion. The galls, on examination, show the presence of mites, various soil fungi and nematodes (*Heterodera* sp) Generally, brown clay soils supporting the natural growth of the plant are found to be infested with nematodes, while dark clay soils are free from them.

(2) *Pyralid Caterpillar Attack*

Pyralid caterpillar (*Glyphodes vertumnalis*) causes appreciable damage to the leaves. The caterpillars roll the leaf and feed on the green matter. Some other caterpillars (*Daphnis nerii* L. and *Deilophola nerii* L.) are also reported to feed on tender leaves, causing defoliation of the plant.

(3) *Cockchafer Grubs Attack*

Cockchafer grubs (*Anomala polita* Blanch.) attack the seedlings about 2 cm below the hypocotyl, resulting in their drying up.

(4) *Leaf-spot Disease*

Leaf-spot disease caused by *Cercospora rauvolfiae* manifests as dark brown coloured spots on the upper surface of the leaf and yellowish brown on the lower surface. The affected leaves turn yellow, become dry and subsequently fall off, resulting defoliation.

(5) *Alternaria Attack*

Alternaria tenuis attacks the leaves resulting in minute, browish or dark coloured circular spots with a yellowish margin on the ventral side of the leaves; there spots enlarge to form prominent dark brown circular lesions. The fungus also affects the flowers and fruits.

(6) *Mosaic Disease*

Mosaic is a common disease found in serpentina field. The primary symptom comprises of vein-banding and gradual yellowing of the leaves, later the leaves curl from the margin to the mid-rib on the abaxial surface and ultimately the leaves drop off. Strict selection of seedlings at the nursery stage helps in avoiding the diseases.

(7) *Die-back Disease*

Die-back disease caused by *Colletotrichum dematium* are found particularly under humid growing conditions. The effected branches may be pruned.

Harvesting

Roots of exploitable size are generally collected 2–3 years after planting. It is reported that the roots dug out in winter (December) in Dehra Dun, when the plants have shed their leaves, are far richer in the total alkaloid content than the roots harvested in August. Roots are dug up, freed from the adhering soil and thoroughly air-dried and packed usually in gunny bags. On air-drying, the moisture content of roots drops to 12–20 percent, but roots containing less than 8 percent of moisture store better; this can be brought about by artificial drying. The root bark constitutes 40–56 percent of the whole roots and contains more alkaloid than the woody portion. Hence care should be taken to keep the bark intact while harvesting.

A light irrigation should be given in advance to facilitate easy digging of roots. The roots may be dug out carefully from the subsoil, manually or by using mould board plough.

Post-harvest Processing

The roots are freed from the adhering soil, washed if necessary and thoroughly air or sun dried till they become brittle and are usually packed in gunny bags or polythene bags.

Yield

Though *R. serpentina* can be propagated by various methods, optimum yield of roots (including thick, thin and fibrous) is obtained when propagaiton is done by seeds. The yield of fresh roots per plant varies widely from 0.1 kg to 4.0 kg. With a spacing of 60 cm × 30 cm and a survival percentage of 80, the total yield of roots in the case of plants raised from seeds works out to about 1,175 kg (air-dry basis) per hectare as compared with 175 kg in the case of plants raised from stem cuttings and 345 kg in the case of plants raised from root cuttings. A yield of 2,200 kg of air-dried roots per hectare has been obained from a 2-year old plantation and 3,300 kg from a 3-year old plantation under irrigated agricultural conditions on sandy clay loam soil.

Medicinal Properties

The root is bitter, acrid, heating, sharp, pungent, anthelmintic and is effective against "tridosha", ulcers, poisonous effects of scropion-stiny and snake-bite.

A decoction of the root is employed in labour to increase uterine contractions.

The juice of the leaves is effective for eye diseases, such as for the removal of opacities of the cornea.

4.20 *Satavari*

Botanical Name

Asparagus recemosus **Willd.**

Indian Names

Bengali–Shatamuli; *Gujarati*–Ekalkanto, Satavari; *Hindi*–Chatwal, Satawar, Satmuli, Shakakul; *Kannada*–Aheruballi, Ashadhi, Majjigegadde, Sipariberuballi; *Marathi*–Asvel, Shatavari, Shatmuli; *Orissi*–Chhotaru, Mohajolo, Sotabori; *Sanskrit*–Satavari; *Tamil*–Ammaikodi, Inli-chedi, Kadumulla, Shimai-shadavari; *Telugu*–Pilli-gaddalu, Toala-gaddalu.

Botanical Family

Liliaceae.

Suitable Places for Growing in India

It is wildly grown in tropical and sub-tropical parts of India including Andamans and ascending in the Himalayas upto an altitude of 1,500 m from Kashmir eastwards.

Botanical Description

Plant

A tall, extensively scandent, much branched, spinous, hardy perennial undershrub with annual woody terete stems.

Roots

Roots tuberous, short rootstock bearing numerous fusiform, succulent tuberous roots 20 –100 cm long and 1–2 cm thick, greyish-white.

Stem

Stems woody, whitish gray or brown armed with strong, straight or recurved spines 5–13 mm long; branchlets triquetrous.

Cladodes

Cladodes more or less acicular, 2–6-nate, falcate,finely acuminate, 1.3–2.5 cm long, leaves reduced to sub-erect or sub-recurved spines.

Flowers

Flowers white, fragrant, small, in solitary or fascicled, simple or branched racemes, 2.5–7 cm long, pedicels 5–5.2 mm long, jointed in the middle, pendulous.

Perianth

Perianth about 3 mm long, white, campanulate, 6 partite.

Androecium

Stamens 3, adnate to the bases of perianth segment; stamens as long as the perianth; anthers oblong, 2-celled, dorsifixed, usually dehiscing longitudinally.

Gynoecium

Ovary 3-celled, tetragynous; style 1; stigmas 3; ovles 2 or more in each overy, anatropous.

Fruit

Berry 5–6 mm diametre, reddish to scarlet globose, trilobed.

Seed: Seeds 2–6; testa black, brittle; embryo dorsal.

Species and Varieties

The plant is rather variable, and three varieties are generally recognized although not distinguished in trade.

(*i*) *Asparagus racemosus* var. *racemosus* with slightly compressed; acuminate, falcate cladodes, and longer, decurved spines, common in partial shades in plains and across upper ghats in Hassan districts in Karnataka.

(*ii*) *Asparagus racemosus* var. *javanicus* Baker (syn. *Asparagopsis javanica* Miq.) has very slender, flexuous racemes with terminal tufts of cladodes and narrower and linear-oblong perianth distributed in the Deccan peninsula, Karnataka, Saurashtra in Gujarat and Bhopal in Madhya Pradesh.

(*iii*) *Asparagus racemosus* var. *subacerosa* Baker. distributed in Sikkim at altitudes of 300–1200 m.

Plant Parts Used

Tuberous roots.

Chemical Component

The plant contains four saponins, *viz.* shatavarin I to IV. Shatavarin IV is a glycoside of sarsasapogenin having two molecules of rhamnose and one molecule of glucose. The saponin, in doses of 20 μg to 500 μg/ml, produces a specific blockade of syntocinon (oxytocin) induced contraction of rat, guineapig and rabbit uteri *in vitro* and *in situ*. It also blocks the uterine spontaneous motility. The bark exhibited anti-bacterial and anti-fungal activities, whereas the aerial parts produce carcinoma of the pharynx in animal trials.

The flowers impart a perfume to the air to a considerable distance. They contain quercetin, rutin (2.5 per cent dry basis) and hyperoside. The mature fruits contain glycosides of quercetin, rutin and hyperoside, also cyanidin-3-galactoside and cyanidin-3-glucorhamnoside. The leaves contain diosgenin and quercetin-3-glucuronide.

Cultivation Procedure

Soil

A. recemosus can be grown in a variety of soils such as sandy loam to red aluviul soil with good drainage system. The plant can be successfully grown in black cotton soil mixed with river sand having pH 7–8.

Climatic Requirements

The plant can be easily grown in sub-tropical and sub-temperate agroclmatic regions upto 1500 mt. It can be grown successfully even in areas, which receives heavy rainfall with high relative humidity. Partial shade (25 per cent) is good for its good growth.

Method of Propagation

A. recemosus can be propagated from seeds and rhizom cuttings and root cutting.

Healthy seeds are sown in well-prepared, raised nursery beds in April–May by broadcasting 5 cm apart to facilitate decay of its hard seed coat by the time monsoon commence. They are then covered with light sand and leaf mould mixture at 1: 1 ratio and regularly watered to keep the bed moist. The seeds germinate within 10–15 days after sowing and the 60 day-old seedlings which are 40–45 cm tall are ready for transplating. It is advisable to transplant the seedlings at a spacing of 60 × 60 cm apart in the field provided bamboo stakes. A plant population of 30,000 plants/ha is considered adequate in moist conditions.

In case of vegetative propagation by root cuttings obtained from adventitious roots are generally used. Pre-soaking the cuttings in liquid cow dung for 24 hour facilitates sprouting. The sprouted saplings are later transferred to the field.

Another type of vegetative propagation may be done by division of rhizomatous disc present at the base of the aerial stem. The rhizomatous disc develop several vegetative buds around the aerial shoots. The disc is divided in such a way that each piece possessed at least two buds along with 2–3 tuberous roots. These pieces are planted, covering the buds with 1 cm of soil followed by irrigation. The sprouting commences in 8–10 days after plantation.

Land Preparation

The land is repeatedly ploughed to 20–30 cm deep and brought to a fine tilth followed by 2–3 harrowings after few days. Grasses, weeds, stubbles and pebbles are to be removed from the field. The land is properly leveled and 40–45 cm broad ridges are prepared for plantation, leaving 15–20 cm furrow space as a channel for irrigation. Pits should be dug with a spacing of 60 cm × 60 cm and the size of the pits should be 30 cm × 30 cm × 30 cm. The pits should be filled with well-decomposed FYM and soil mixture. Groundnut cake, bone-meal, rapeseed cake and vermicompost are also beneficial for plant growth. To remove the mites and nematods from the field, prior application of neem cake is recommended at the doses of 7–12 kg/ha.

Planting

With the onset of monsoon, the saplings are planted in the pits. The pits are gap filled one month after planting.

Manuring

The plant responds very well to organic manure. For the commerical cultivation, 20 tonns of well-rotten FYM should be applied as basal dressing. During 2nd and 3rd year, FYM is spread in the root zone and mixed well with soil.

Irrigation

The crop should be irrigated fortnightly in summer and winter seasons. There is no need of irrigation during rainy season.

Intercultural Measures

The plant requires staking for its proper growth. The stakes should be infixed vertically and horizontally within 3rd month of planting.

Two weedings are necessary during the rainy months followed by one in next 4 months.

After the application of FYM to the beds, earthing-up should be done.

Intercropping

Asparagus recemosus may be planted as an intercrop in eucalyptus, coconut, arecanut plantation in different parts of the country.

Crop Protection Measures

This plant is very hardy in nature and is free from any pest and diseases of serious nature.

Harvesting

The roots of *A. recemosus* are borne in a compact bunch and are fleshy, and spindle-shaped. They are silvery white or light ash-coloured externally and white internally, more or less smooth when fresh, developing longitudinal wrinkles when dry. They lack a well-marked colour, but are sweet and bitter in taste.

The roots are harvested after 40 months of transplantation during winter season. At the time of harvesting, the stems are cut close to the ground and roots are dug up.

Post-harvest Processing

Harvested roots are cleaned in water and peeled off with the help of sharp knife immediately after harvesting. It is observed that in case the roots are not peeled off within a few days, it is a bit difficult to remove the skin from them. In such condition the roots are kept in boiling water for about 10 minutes, followed by cold-water treatment facilitate peeling.

After removing the skin, the roots are cut transversely into small pieces and dried in shade. They are then graded and packed in gunny bags.

Yield

The average yield of dried root are 8–8.5 tonnes/ha.

Medicinal Properties

The roots are bitter sweet; oleaginous, cooling, indigestible, appetiser; alterative, stomachic, tonic, aphrodisiac, galactagogue, astringent to the bowels and useful in dysentery, tumours, inflammations, biliousness, blood diseases and the eye, throat complaints, tuberculosis, leprosy, epilepsy, night blindness etc.

The root is used as a refrigerant, demulcent, diuretic, aphrodisiac antipasmodic, alterative, antidiarrhoeatic and anti-dysenteric. It is used as a demulcent in veterinary medicine.

4.21 Sweet Flag (Syn. Calamus Sweet Root)

Botanical Name

Acorus calamus Linn.

Indian Names

Bengali–Bach; *Hindi*–Bach, Gorbacc; *Gujarati*–Vekhand; *Marathi*–Vekhand; *Kannada*–Baje; *Malayali*–Vayampa; *Tamil*–Vashambu; *Telugu*–Vasa; *Assamis*–Bach.

Botanical Family

Araceae.

Suitable Places for Growing in India

It can be cultivated throughout India, ascending to an altitude of 2,200 m in the Himalayas. The major cultivators states are Karnataka, Kashmir, Manipur, Arunachal Pradesh, Meghalaya and the foot hills of Himalayas.

Botanical Description

Plant

Aromatic marsh herbs, rootstock as thick as the middle finger, creeping and branching.

Stem

Absent.

Leaves

Leaves distichous, ensiform, base equitant, 0.9–1.8 m by 1.7–3.8 cm, bright green, acute, thickened in the middle, margins waved, nerves parallel.

Flowers

Spathe the ensiform continuation of the leaf-like peduncle, 15–75 cm long, pedicel (formed of connate pedicel and spathe) 3.8–3.2 cm broad. Spadix sessile, cylindric, dense-flowered, flowering upwards, 5–10 by 1.3–2.2 cm diam.; obtuse, slighthly curved, green.

Calyx

Sepals 6, orbicular, concave tips, incurved, as long as the ovary, scarious.

Corolla

Absent.

Androecium

Stames 6, filaments linear flat; anther reniform, yellow, cells confluent above, slits entrorse.

Gynoecium

Ovary conical, 2–3-celled; stigma minute; ovules many, pendulous from the top of each cell, orthotropous.

Fruit

Berries, few seeded, turbinate, prismatic, top pyramidal.

Seeds

Seeds oblong, micropyle often fimbriate, albumen fleshy, embryo axile.

Species and Varieties

Acorus gramineus Soland. ex. Ait., a Japanese species is occassionally cultivated within Sikkim upto an altitude of 1,800 m and in Khasi hills up to 1,500 m.

Plant Parts Used

Rhizome.

Chemical Component

The roots, rhizomes and leaves contain a brownish volatile oil which is known as calamus oil having good aroma and sweetness. The important constituents of the Indian calamus oil are asarone (8.2 per cent) and its β-isomer, calamenol (5.0 per cent), calamene (0.4 per cent), calamenone (1.0 per cent), methyl eugenol (1.0 per cent), eugenol (0.3 per cent), α-pinene and camphene (0.2 per cent) Besides these, trace amount of palmitic acid heptylic acid, butyric acid, asaronaldehyde, calamol, calamone, azulene, acorone, calarene, calacone, calacorene, acorenone, acolamone, isoacolamone, epishyobunone, shyobunone, isoshyobunone, acoragermacrone, isocalamendiol, preisocalamendiol, elemene, caryophyllene,calamenene, cadalene also found in the rhizomatous roots of calamus.

Roots produce choline (0.26 per cent) and acoric acid. Tannins, mucilage and calcium oxalate are also present in roots.

Cultivation Procedure

Soil

The plant is grown well in clayey loam and alluvial soils along river banks. Sweet flag is grown in water its wild state but may be cultivated in almost any good, but fairly moist soil. It is generally grown in areas where paddy is grown.

Climatic Requirements

The plant is hardy and is grown in tropical and sub-tropical climates. It prefers an area having good and well-distributed rainfall throughout the year and grows well in marshy and moist places.

Method of Propagation

The live ends of the growing tops of the previous crop consist of the planting materials. At harvest, the mature part of the rhizome is cut off, which is marketed and the tender part formed by the growing end is used for replanting. The planting materials can be set at once or stored for one to two weeks, by covering it with straw or dried leaves. When required to be stored for a long time, these can be stored in open pits.

Land Preparation

The field is laid out exactly as is done in rice. After ploughing with 400 tonns of Fym/ha, the field is watered heavily, ploughed again and impounded like rice field. Then it is left as such for a few days and puddled. After that, it is leveled and planted.

Planting

The best season of planting is spring, *i.e.* March–April, although planting may be done almost any time of the year provided plenty of sunshine is available at harvest time to dry the rhizomes.

Sweet flag is planted maintaining a spacing of 30 cm × 30 cm. The rhizome pieces are pressed into the soft mud at a depth of about 5 cm inside the soil leaving the leafy portions well above the ground. The rhizomes are set in such a way that the plants in the second row comes in-between the first row and not opposite to it. The field should be flooded with 5 cm deep water after planting.

Manuring

Green manuring before planting is very good. In absence of that, 15 tonns of compost/ha should be applied.

Irrigation

The field should be regularly irrigated with about 5 cm water to stand at the beginning. Later, the water level should be increased to 10 cm as the plant grows.

Intercultural Measures

Regular weeding is no doubt, a necessity to the crop. In all, eight weedings are given and at each weeding, the growing plants are lightly pressed down into the soil with feet.

Intercropping

The crop may be grown as an intercrop with *Asterocanthus longifolia*.

Crop Protection Measures

This crop is virtually free from the attack of any pest or disease of serious nature. However, in some area the following pest may attack the crop.

(1) Mealy Bug Attack

The pest attack the shoot and roots of young and mature plants.

Harvesting

The crop becomes ready for harvest after an year of planting. For harvesting, the field is allowed to dry partially so that sufficient moisture is retained to facilitate the necessary deep digging. The leaves starting turning yellow and drying are indicative of harvest-maturity. The rhizomes are produced at a depth of 60 cm and these become 30–60 cm long. Harvesting should be done carefully. On digging out the plants, the rhizomes are removed and the tops kept for the next planting.

Post-harvest Processing

After harvest, the rhizomes are cut into short lengths of 5–7.5 cm and all the adhering fibrous roots are removed. The pieces are then thoroughly washed and dried in the sun. The dried materials are put into gunny bags and rubbed to make them free from of leafy scales.

Yield

The yield of rhizome may be 10–12 tonns/ha when proper cultivation management is followed.

Medicinal Properties

The rhizome has laxative, diuretic, carminative and anthelmintic properties. It improves appetite, voice, throat and is useful for diseases of the mouth, abdominal pains, inflammation, fevers, epilepsy, bronchitis, delirium, hysteria, dysentery, tumours, thirst, loss of memory, rat-bite, worms in the ear etc. It is also used in kidney trouble, hepatitis, toothache, leucoderma and as a brain tonic.

The root has been employed in medicine since long past. It is successfully used in intermittent fevers, even when chinchona bark has failed. Besides, it is also a useful adjunct to bitter and stomachic infusions and is much valued by the Manipuris, especially in the treatment of coughs or sore-throats. For this purpose, a small piece is chewed by them for few minutes.

Bach is especially used to allay distressing cough. A small piece of the dried rhizome kept in the mouth acts better than many cough lozenges. On doing so, a warm sensation is produced in the mouth with a beneficial discharge of salvia.

The root is extremely useful for dysentery and in bronchial afflictions.

4.22 Thyme-leaved Gratiola

Botanical Name

Bacopa monnieri (Linn) Wettst.

Indian Names

Bengali–Brahmi-sak, Jalanimba; *Hindi*–Barambhi, Bhrahmi; *Kannada*–Nirubrahmi; Mal., *Marathi* & *Tamil*–Neer-brahmi; *Sanskrit*–Brahmi, Brahmacharini, Nira-brahmi; *Telugu*–Sambrani-chettu, *Orissi*–Krishnaparni.

Botanical Family

Scrophulariaceae.

Suitable Places for Growing in India

It can be grown in marshy places throughout India, ascending to an altitude of 1,320 m. It is found in Uttar Pradesh, Punjab, Haryana, Bihar, West Bengal, Tamil Nadu, Kerala, Karnataka, foot hills of Himachal Pradesh and Uttaranchal.

Botanical Description

Plant

A small creeping succulent herb, branches profusely and rooting at the nodes.

Stem

Stem obtuse-angular, soft, much branched.

Leaves

Succulent leaves are sessile, decussate, short petioled, oblong-cuneate to obovate, 1.0–2.5 cm by 0.4–1.0 cm, lower opposite and the upper are alternate.

Flower

Flower solitary, axillary, white or purple-tinged; zygomorphic, bisexual, hypogynous, bractate.

Calyx

Sepals 5, more or less deeply 5 partite; imbricate.

Corolla

Petals-5, personate, imbricate; white with tinged with purple and yellow.

Androecium

Stamens 4, didynamous, epipetalous, inserted, anther-cells contiguous.

Gynoecium

Carpels-2, medianly placed; ovary superior, usually 2-celled with numerous anatropous ovules on axile placentation; stigma simple; style-terminal.

Fruit

Ovoid capsul.

Seed

Seed albuminous, embryo straight or slightly curved.

Species and Varieties

At present there is no named or certified varieties under this crop under cultivation.

Plant Parts Used

Whole plant.

Chemical Component

The herb contains the alkaloids brahmine, herpestine and a mixture of three bases. Brahmine is highly toxic when administered at a dose of 0.5 mg/kg bod;· wt. of cat, it produces a fall in blood pressure. In therapeutic doses, it resembles strychnine. The herb also contains the saponins, monnierin; hersaponin, bacoside A and bacoside B. Moninierin, on hydrolysis, gave glucose, arabinose and an aglycone whereas, bacosides A and B gave glucose, arabinose and bacogenins A_1, A_2, A_3 and A_4; bacogenins A_1 and A_2 are epimers, and A_4 is an ebelin lactone. Bacosides A and B possess haemolytic activity. Other constituents present in the plant are D-mannitol, betulic acid, β-sitosterol, stigmasterol and its esters. Heptacosane, octacosane, nonacosane, triacontane, hentriacontane, dotriacontane, nicotine, 3-formyl-4-hydroxy-2H-pyran ($C_6H_6O_3$), luteolin, and its glucoside. The presence of α-alanine, aspartic acid, glutamic acid and serine is also found.

Analysis of the leaves and stalks of the plants give moisture (88.4 per cent), protein (2.1 per cent), fat (0.6 per cent), carbohydrates (5.9 per cent), crude fibre (1.05 per cent), ash (1.9 per cent), calcium 202.0 mg/100 g, phosphorus 16.0 mg/100 g, iron 7.8 mg/100 g, ascorbic acid 63.0 mg/100 g; nicotinic acid 0.3 mg/100 g, and energy 38 kcal/100 g.

Cultivation Procedure

Soil

The plant can be grown under varying type of soil and climatic conditions. It grows quite well in poorly drained soil also and in marshy land.

Climatic Requirements

The plant thrives well under sub-tropical condition. The plant grow faster of temperatures (33–40°C) with high relative humidity (65–80 per cent) and is cultivated in summer to rainy season.

Method of Propagation

The plants are propagated vegetatively by stem cuttings. Stem cutting which are about 4–5 cm long and each containing few leaves, nodes and roots serve as ideal planting materials. These can be obtained by cutting from the mother plants making small pieces.

Land Preparation

The land is prepared by repeated ploughing and levelling to bring to a fine tilth. About 25 tonnes of FYM per hectare is mixed well with the soil at the time of the last ploughing. The land is laid out into plots of convenient sizes with provision of irrigation channels for easy management.

The land should be irrigated a day before planting for successful establishment of plant cuttings.

Planting

The cuttings are transplanted in wet soil at a spacing of 40 cm × 40 cm. Heavy irrigation should be done immediately after planting. Ideally, the plants should be transplanted in March–June and are allowed to grow and proliferate through hot and humid months of the monsoon till September, after which harvesting may be done.

Manuring

Bhrahmi responds well to the application of well-decomposed FYM @ 15–20 tonnes per hectare area of land at the time of field preparation.

Irrigation

Immediately after transplanting, irrigation is essential for successful survival of the plants. Subsequently the fields are irrigated by flooding as per requirement usually at every 7–8 days.

Intercultural Measures

Initially, hand-weeding is required at every 5–20 days interval. Later, as the plant proliferates and form a dense mat of vegetation, weeding may be done sporadically as and when needed.

Crop Protection Measures

Brahmi is usually not attacked by pests and disease of serious nature.

Harvesting

The plants should be harvested between October–November. After that, there is loss of plant biomass and the *bacoside* yield. The plant can also be maintained in perennial state with two harvests in a year of which the first one should be done in June and the other, after the monsoon *i.e.*, in October.

Cutting in such a way that the upper-4–5 cm portions of the stem from the base are removed and the rest parts left for subsequent regeneration can ideally harvest the plant.

Post-harvest Processing

The plants can be dried in a conventional manner by spreading on the ground in open sun or partial shade. Alternatively, they can be dried at 80°C in hot-air-oven for 30 minutes immediately after harvest for a higher retention of *bacoside-A* content of the dried herbs. After this, they can be further air-dried by spreading on the ground at room temperature or in the oven at 37°C.

The dry material should be cleaned and made free from any external matter. The dry material should be stored in a cool and dry room, packed in gunny bag or boxes, having concrete flooring and away from walls.

Precautions need to be taken to avoid infestation with fungi and insects.

Yield

Under favourable and well agro-management condition, 4–4.25 tonns per hectare of dry herb may be obtained.

Medicinal Properties

Brahmi has a remarkable effect in sharpening of memory. Besides that, in nervous disorders like epilepsy respiratory and urinary tract infections, rheumatism and many other infections, it is used.

4.23 Trailing eclipta

Botanical Names

Eclipta alba Hassk., *E. prostrate.*

Indian Names

Sanskrit–Bhringaraja, Kesaraja, Ajagara; *Hindi*–Bhangra, Mochkand, Babri; *Bengali*–Kesuti, Keshukti, Keshori; *Marathi*–Bhringuraja, Maka; *Gujarati*–Bhangra, Kaluganthi, Dodhak, Kalobhangro; *Tamil*–Garuga, Kayanthakara; *Kannada*–Garagadasoppy; *Malayali*–Kyonni; *Orissi*–Kesarda.

Botanical Family

Compositae.

Suitable Places for Growing in India

This plant is a common weed in moist situation throughout India, ascending up to 6,000 ft on the hills.

Botanical Description

Plant

Annual, erect or prostrate, branched, often rooting at the nodes.

Stem

Stem and branches strigose with appressed white hairs.

Leaves

Leaves sessile, 2.5–7.5 cm long, variable in breadth, usually oblong-lanceolate, subentire, acute or subacute, sparsely stringose with appressed hairs on both sides, base tapering.

Inflorescence

Heads 6–8 mm diam., solitary or 2 together on unequal axillary peduncles. Involucral bracts about 8, ovate, abtuse or acute, herbaceous, strigose with appressed white hairs. Receptacle flat or somewhat convex, the paleae narrow, enclosing several flowers, the inner most very narrow or 0. Ray flowers female, sub-2seriate, fertile or sterile, white or yellow; disc flowers hermaphrodites, fertile.

Corolla

Corolla of ray-flowers ligulate, the ligule small, spreading, scarcely as long as the bracts, not toothed, white.

Corolla of disk-flowers regular, tubular, the limb shortly 4–5 fid, often 4-toothed, pappus absent, except occationally very minute teeth on the top of the achene.

Androecium

Stamens 5, inserted on the corolla and alternate with its segments; filaments usually free above; anther bases obtuse, subentire, 2-celled, introrse, cohering into a tube which sheaths the style.

Gynoecium

Ovary 1-celled; ovule solitary, erect, anatropous, style-arms flattened, terminated by short or thiangular obtuse appendages.

Fruit

Achenes cuneate, compressed and with a narrow wing, covered with warty excrescences.

Seed

Seed erect; testa membranous, exalbuminous; embryo straight; cotyledons plano-convex; radicle short.

Species and Varieties

Wedelia chinensis Merrill. (syn. *W. calendulacea* Less.) is commonly used, to some extent, vicariously for *E. alba*.

Plant Parts Used

Whole plant.

Chemical Component

Chemically it is composed of roal and ecliptine bases. An element called wedelolactone is also found in yellow *Bhringaraj*.

The plant content 0.078 per cent nicotine on dry basis. The leaves contain stigmasterol and α-ter-thienylmethanl; small amount of 2-formyl-terthienyl; wedelolactone, de-Me-wedelolacton and its 7–0-glucoside. Aerial parts of Egyption plant is reported to be contained β-amyrin, wedelolactone, luteolin-7-glucoside, phytosterol A and its glucosides.

Cultivation Procedure

Soil

The plant can be grown under varying type of soil and climatic conditions. It grows quite well in poorly drained soil also and in marshy land.

Climatic Requirements

The plant thrives well under sub-tropical condition. The plant grow faster of temperatures (33–40°C) with high relative humidity (65–80 per cent) and is cultivated in summer to rainy season.

Method of Propagation

The plants are propagated vegetatively by stem cuttings. Stem cutting which are about 4–5 cm long and each containing few leaves, nodes and roots serve as ideal planting materials. These can be obtained by cutting from the mother plants making small pieces.

Land Preparation

The land is prepared by repeated ploughing and leveling to bring to a fine tilth. About 25 tonns of FYM per hectare is mixed well with the soil at the time of the last ploughing. The land is laid out into plots of convenient sizes with provision of irrigation channels for easy management.

The land should be irrigated a day before planting for successful establishment of plant cuttings.

Planting

The cuttings are transplanted in wet soil at a spacing of 40 cm × 40 cm. Heavy irrigation should be done immediately after planting. Ideally, the plants should be transplanted in March–June and are allowed to grow and proliferate through hot and humid months of the monsoon till September, after which harvesting may be done.

Manuring

Bhringaraja responds well to the application of well-decomposed FYM @ 15–20 tonns per hectare area of land at the time of field preparation.

Irrigation

Immediately after transplanting, irrigation is essential for successful survival of the plants. Subsequently the fields are irrigated by flooding as per requirement usually at every 7–8 days.

Intercultural Measures

Initially, hand-weeding is required at every 5–20 days interval. Later, as the plant proliferates and form a dense mat of vegetation, weeding may be done sporadically as and when needed.

Crop Protection Measures

Bhringaraja is usually not attacked by pests and disease of serious nature.

Harvesting

The leaves, stems and roots may be harvested after two months of plantation.

They can be ideally harvested by cutting in such a way so that the upper portion of the stem 4–5 cm from the base are removed and rest left for subsequent regeneration.

Leaves may be harvested 6–8 times in year.

Post-harvest Processing

The plants can be dried in a conventional manner by spreading on the ground in open sun or partial shade. Alternatively, they can be dried at 80°C in hot-air-oven for 30 minutes immediately after harvest. After this, they can be further air-dried by spreading on the ground at room temperature or in the oven at 37°C.

The dry material should be cleaned and made free from any external matter. The dry material should be stored in a cool and dry room, packed in gunny bag or boxes, having concrete flooring and away from walls.

Precautions need to be taken to avoid infestation with fungi and insects.

Yield

Under favourable condition 3–3.5 tonnes per hectare of dry herb may be obtained.

Medicinal Properties

The plant has a bitter hot sharp dry taste; faltening, alterative, anthelmintic, alexipharmic; good for hair, eyes, teeth etc.; cures inflammations, hernias, eye diseases, "kapha" and "vata", bronchitis, asthma, leucoderma, anaemia, diseases of the heart and the skin, itching, night-blindness, syphilis; used to prevent abortion and miscarriage, and for uterine pains after delivery.

It is largely used as a tonic and deobstruent in hepatic and splenic enlargements, and in various chronic skin diseases. There is a popular opinion that the herb taken internally and applied topically turns the hair black.

The fresh juice of the leaves is rubbed on the shaven scalp for promoting the growth of hair.

In Maharastra, the people use the juice in combination with aromatics, as a tonic and deobstruent, and give two drops of it with eight drops of honey to new-born child, suffering from catarrh.

The fresh plant is applied with sesamum oil in elephantiasis, and the expressed juice in diseases of the liver and in dropsy. When used in large doses, it acts as an emetic. It is anudyne and absorbent, and relieves headache when applied with a little oil.

There are two varieties of the plant which are the yellow flowered and the white flowered. The former variety has thicker leaves which are extensively used in catarrhal jaundice. The fresh leaves are ground and a lump of the size of a lime is administered early in the morning in sour curd or butter milk.

The juice of the leaves is febrifuge and the root is given to relieve the scalding of urine.

The plant is considered as an astringent in China, and is used for checking haemorrhages and fluxes and strengthening of the gums.

The plant is much used to cure asthma and bronchitis in Indo-China.

4.24 Winter cherry

Botanical Name

Withania somnifera **(Linn.) Dunal**

Indian Names

Sanskrit–Ashwagandha; *Hindi*–Punir, Asgandh; *Bengali*–Ashvagandha; *Marathi*–Askandha Tilli; *Gujarati*–Ghodakun,

Ghoda, Asoda, Asan; *Telugu*–Pulivendram, Panneru-gadda, Panneru; *Tamil*–Amukkura, Amkulang, Amukkuram-kilangu, Amulang-kalung (root), Aswagandhi; *Kannada*–Viremaddlinagadde, Pannaeru, Aswagandhi, Kiremallinagida.

Botanical Family

·Solanaceae.

Suitable Places for Growing in India

W. somnifera is found wild in grazing grounds in Mandsaur and the forest lands of Bastar district of Madhya Pradesh, all over the foothills of the Punjab and Himachal Pradesh and western Uttar Pradesh in the Himalayas.

The crop is cultivated mainly in the drier parts of Manasa, Neemuch and Jawad tehsils of the Mandsour District of Madhya Pradesh in Punjab, Sind, Rajasthan, south India and Karnataka specially in Mysore district.

Botanical Description

Plant

A branched erect under shurb 0.3–1.5 m high; branches terete, usually clothed with mealy whitish, stellate hairy tomentum.

Roots

Root stout, fleshy, whitish brown, tapering.

Stem

Stem erect, stout, branched.

Leaves

Leaves 5–10 by 2.5–5 cm, ovate, subacute, entire, more or less minutely stellately pubescent, base acute to cuneate; main nerves about 6 pairs, stout, conspicuous; petioles 6–13 mm long, stellately tomentose beneath. Leaves in floral region smallar and opposite.

Flowers

Flowers insconspicuous greenish or lurid yellow, axilary, usually about 5–25 together in a sessile or nearly sessile umbellate cyme; pedicels 0.4–0.6 mm long.

Calyx

Calyx 5.5 mm long in flower, stellately tomentose; teeth 2.5 mm long, linear acute, from a deltoid base.

Corolla

Corolla 5.8 mm long, divided rather more than ½ way down; lobes lanceolate, acute, pubescent outside.

Androecium

Stamens 5, filaments 3 mm long, slender, glabrous; anthers broadly elliptic (almost orbicular), 1.25 mm long, attached to corolla tube and bear erect anthors which form a close colume or one around the style. Pollen production is very poor.

Gynoecium

Ovary glabrous, style glabrous, two celled, single styled and bilobed stigma.

Fruit

Brery globose, smooth, 6–7 mm diameter, enclosed in the inflated membranous, persistent calyx which reaches more than 2.5 cm diam., calyx slightly 5-angled, pointed with the connivent calyx-teeth and scurfy-pubescent outside. The fruits turn orange-red in colour when they mature.

Seed

Seeds 2.5 mm diam., yellow, somewhat scurfy, reniform in shape.

Species and Varieties

WS 10, WS 12, WS 14, WS 16, WS 19, WS 20 and WS 22 are some of released varieties. WS 20 or Jawahar Asgandh is recommended for general cultivation of all parts of India. Besides these *W. congulans* is also cultivated in many parts of India.

Plant Parts Used

Roots.

Chemical Component

Roots

The roots have a short and uneven fracture, a strong odour and mucilaginous bitter and acrid taste. The young tuberous roots and older roots have distinct macroscopic and microscopic characters. The drug is official as a sedative in the Pharmacopoeia of India. The powdered drug is grayish with pungent odour and acid taste. It is characterized by the presence of a large number of starch-grains, cork-cells, cortical and xylem-parenchyma, tracheids, vessels and wood-fibres.

The pharmacological activity of the roots is attributed to the presence of several alkaloids. The total alkaloid content of the Indian roots has been reported to vary between 0.13 and 0.31 percent, though much higher yields (up to 4.3 per cent) have been recorded elesewhere. The wide variations in the yields might be due to factors, such as methods of isolation used, variability in species, environment, and wild or cultivated forms. The yield may also vary due to extensive resinification of the fractions representing total or separated alkaloids (resulting in the loss of alkaloid) and the presence of steroidal material as a major component positively reacting on modified Dragendorff's reagent.

Many biochemically heterogeneous alkaloids have been reported in the roots. In all, 13 Dragendorff positive components have been obtained chromatographically. They include cuscohygrine (pyridine derivative), hygrine (one pyrrolidine and one piperidine) tropine, pseudotropine, anaferine and its *dl*-form, *isopelletierine* (piperidine derivative) and 3-tropyltigloate; other components remain unidentified. The presence of nicotine in the Indian roots, reported in an earlier work could not be confirmed. The same alkaloids are present in both the wild and the cultivated forms of *W. somnifera*.

In addition to the alkaloids, the roots are reported to contain starch, reducing sugars, hentriacontane, glycosides, dulcitol, withaniol (0.08 per cent) Withaniol was later found to be a mixture of two withanolides, of which the major component was 5,20α-(R)-dihydroxy-6α, 7α-epoxy-l-oxo-(5α)-witha-2, 24-dienolide, and the minor component remained unidentified. The free amino acids identified in the roots include aspartic acid, glycine, tyrosine, alanine, proline, tryptophan, glutamic acid and cystine. The roots of South-African origin yielded a small amount of a light brown, pungent volatile oil.

Leaves

W. somnifera shows a chemical variability, particularly noticeable in the case of leaves. The leaves of the plant from different habitats contain different withanolides. Three different chemotypes of *W. somnifera* have been found to occur in Israel; they show a definite geographical distribution, but no morphological differences. The difference between these chemotypes resides in the substitution pattern of the withanolides. The plants of these chemotypes raised from the seeds in a uniform nursery showed the same pattern of withanolides as those taken from their natural habitat. There seems to be a greater concentration of withanolides in the leaves at the stage of maximum vegetative development.

The plants raised in Israel from Jamnagar (Gujarat) seeds contained only three withanolides: withaferin A; 5α, 17α-dihydroxy-l-oxo-6α, 7α-epoxy-witha-2, 24-dienolide; and a minor withanolide ($C_{28}H_{38}O_5$) The former two withanolides from Delhi region. A different pattern of withanolides was found in the South-African plants. Somnirol and Somnitol, obtained earlier from the leaves in South Africa and in West Bengal, are in all probability withanolides; however, no mention has been made of these compounds in the recent investigations.

In addition to withanolides, the leaves from Delhi region contained five unidentified alkaloids (yield, 0.09 per cent), glycosides, glucose and many free amino acids. Occurrence of chlorogenic acid, condensed tannins (also in the stems), and flavonoid is reported elsewhere.

Withaferin A–Withaferin A is the most important of the withanolides isolated so far, to which the curative properties of the leaves are attributed. It has been receiving a good deal of attention because of its antibiotic and antitumour activities. The patented insaturated lactone-antibiotic, obtained from the Indian plant, is identical with withaferin A. For its sepration, the leaves are extracted with cold alcohol; the extract is purified and dried, and finally crystallized from aqueous alcohol (yield, 0.18 per cent air-dry basis) The yield of this compound from the South-African plants is reported to be as high as 0.86 percent. Withaferin A can also be obtained from the leaves by methanolic extraction, fractionation and chromatographic separation. It is insoluble in water and is administered in the form of suspension.

Cultivation Procedure

Soil

W. somnifera can be grown successfully in sandy loam or light-red soils with good organic matter and drainage system. A soil pH range from 7.5–8 is best for its good yield. It can also be grown in medium fertile soil with little care where other crops are unsuitable.

Climatic Requirements

This plant prefers subtropical and low rainfal regions. It can be cultivated between 600–1200 m altitude to plains. It is grown as a long-duration winter annual (240 days) on marginal lands in Madhya Pradesh as a rainfed crop. The sub-tropical areas receiving 500–750 mm rainfall are suitable for cultivation of this rainfed crop. The crop requires dry season during its growing period. Temperature between 20°C to 35°C is most suitable for its cultivation. 1–2 late winter showers favour its good root development.

Method of Propagation

The plant is generally propagated from seeds for commercial purpose. It may be grown by directly sowing the seeds in the field as well as by raising seedlings and transplating them.

The direct sowing method, the seeds are sown directly in the field by broadcasting in lines. The time of sowing in the field is determined by the onset of monsoon as it is mainly cultivated as a rainfed crop. After receiving one or two pre-monsoon shower the field is prepared and seeds are sown during the second week of July. A seed rate of 10 –12 kg/ha is required for this method of planting.

In nursery raising and transplanting method seeds are sown broadcast in well-prepared raised nursery beds just before the onset of rainy season. The seeds are usually sown about lines spaced at 5 cm and 1–3 cm deep in June–July in nursery. Seeds are covered with a mixture of light soil and leaf mould. A light irrigation after sowing results a good germination. About 5 kg of seeds are sufficient to provide seedlings for an area of one hectare field. The germination starts within 6–7 days of seed-sowing and in about 10 days after sowing it is completed.

Land Preparation

The plant is usually grown in fields which are not well covered by irrigation systems. Mainly *W. somnifera* is grown in marginal fields where profitable crops can not be grown.

After receiving two to three showers the field is thoroughly pulverized by repeatedly ploughing, disking or harrowing. Then the field is leveled and divided into plots of convenient sizes.

Planting

25–35 day-old seedlings attaining good height are transplanted in the field in 60 cm wide furrows at 60 cm apart.

Manuring

This crop does not require heavy doses of manure. In Madhya Pradesh, no fertilizers are applied and the crop is cultivated on only soil original fertility. However 250 kg of well-rotten FYM per hectare of land is a recommendation from the experts.

Irrigation

Light irrigation just after transplantation helps the seedlings for well establishment in the field. There is no requirement of additional irrigation if there is good rainfal at regular intervals. But if there is a long dry season, life saving irrigation may be applied if required. Excessive rainfal is harmful to the plant.

Intercultural Measures

The seeds sown by broadcasting or in the line in furrows should be thinned out by hand at 25–30 days after sowing to maintain a plant population of about 3.5–6 lakh plants/ha. However, the plant density to be followed may depend on the nature and fertility of the soil. On the marginal land the population in kept high.

Weeding cum hoeing by hand at 25–30 days interval helps to control the weeds effectively and a better root growth.

Intercropping

The plant may be grown as an intercrop with any tree plantation.

Crop Protection Measures

The plant is hardy in nature and very few insects and diseases generally attack the crop. However, in some area some attack of pest and diseases are found. They are as follows:

(1) Shoot Borer Aattack

Young plants are been affected from this caterpillar.

(2) *Mites Attack*

Mites damages the crop by cutting off the roots. They may be effectively controlled by application of neem-cake or neem-based pesticides at the time of land preparation.

(3) *Seed Rotting Disease*

This is a common diseases affecting *Aswagandha* plantation. Their incidence may be minimise by 24 hrs treating the seeds with bio-fungicides before sowing.

(4) *Seedling Blight Disease*

Seeldings in seedbed are affected in this disease. This disease may reduce the plant population drastically. Drainage should be ensured in the beds.

(5) *Leaf Blight Disease*

Alternaria species attack the young and mature plants causing the disease. Poor drainage system helps the disease to rapidly spread among the population.

(6) *Die-back Disease*

The other disease reported on this crop is die-back or seedling mortality. When the weather is highly humid and the temperature is high, seedling mortality becomes serious. The disease can be minimised by using healthy seedlings in the field.

Harvesting

The plants start flowering and fruiting from December onwards. Harvesting starts from January and continues till March at 150 to 180 days after sowing. The maturity of the crop is judged by the drying of leaves and the berries turning yellow-red in colour.

The entire plants are uprooted for roots, which are separated from aerial parts by cutting the stem 1–2 cm above the crown.

Berries are hand plucked from the dried plants are threshed to obtain the seeds.

Post-harvest Processing

The uprooted roots are cut into smaller pieces of 7–10 cm to facilitate drying in the sum. Some times they are dried as a whole. The dried whole roots undergo cleaning, trimming and grading before storing. They are often beaten with a club to remove the adhering soil and the thin lateral roots and rootlets. The main tap root may be cut into transverse pieces. Lateral branches, root crown and stem portion remains on roots are carefully trimmed with the help of knife.

The dried roots are then carefully hand-graded and stored into four grades, based on the thickness and uniformity of pieces.

A Grade

Root pieces upto 7 cm in length, solid and 1–1.5 cm diameter, and they should be brittle and pure white inside.

B Grade

Root pieces upto 5 cm in length, solid, with a diameter of less than 1 cm, the roots should be brittle and white inside.

C Grade

Root pieces upto 3–4 cm in length, side branches solid, with a diameter of 1 cm or less.

Lower Grade

Small root pieces, semi-solid, very thin and yellowish inside.

These roots are wrapped in gunny bags and stored in well-ventilated cool godowns for a long period without loss in quality.

Yield

An average yield of about 5–7 q/ha of dried roots and 50–75 kg/ha of seed can be obtained from a well-managed commercial field.

Medicinal Properties

The tuber is bitter, sharp and acrid in taste. It is also an aphrodisiac and is anthelmintic and is useful in "vata" and "kapha", inflamations, psoriasis, bronchitis, asthma, consumption, ulcers, scabies, marasmus of childred, insomnia, senile debilty; alexipharmic.

The root is regarded as a tonic, alterative and aphrodisiac and is used in consumption, emaciation of children, debility from old age, rheumatism etc. It has also narcotic, diuretic and deobstruent properties.

In Rajasthan area, the root is of much use in rheumatism and dyspepsia.

In Punjab, it is used for lumber pains for increasing sex desire.

In Sind, the root is used to induce abortion.

The ground root and bruised leaves are employed as a local application to carbuncles, ulcers and painful swellings. The leaves are very bitter, and are given in infusion in fever.

The fruit is diuretic. The seeds are employed to coagulate milk. They are diuretic and hypnotic.

4.25 Yellow-Berried Nightshade

Botanical Name

Solanum xanthocarpum **Schrad. Wendl.**

Indian Names

Sanskrit–Kantikari, Nidigadhika; *Hindi*–Kateli, Katai, Ringani; *Bengali*–Kantikari; *Marathi*–Bhuiringani; *Gujarati*–Bhoyaringani; *Telugu*–Pinnamulaka, Nelamulaka, Vankuda; *Tamil & Malayali*–Kandankattiri; *Orissi*–Bheji Begun, Ankranti; *Punjabi*–Kandyali, Mahori, Warumba.

Botanical Family

Solanaceae.

Suitable Places for Growing in India

This Plant can be grown throughout India in dry parts, up to an elevation of 2,100 m.

Botanical Description

Plant

A very prickly diffuse, bright-green perennial herb up to 1.2 m tall somewhat woody at the base.

Root

Root is 3–5 cm long and 1.5–6 mm thick, dull-grayish in colour with a soft, fibrous fracture.

Stem

Stem somewhat zigzag; branches numerous, the younger ones

clothed with dense, stellate tomentum; prickles compressed, straight, yellow, glabrous and shinning, often exceeding 1.3 cm long.

Leaves

Leaves 5–10 by 2.5–5.7 cm, ovate or elliptic, sinuate or subpinnatifid, obtuse or subacute, stellately hairy on the both sides (especially so beneath), sometimes becoming nearly glabrous in age, armed on the midrib and often on the nerves with long yellow sharp prickles, spine 1 cm long, straight, base usually rounded and unequal sided; petioles 1.3–2.5 cm long, stellately hairy and prickly.

Flowers

Flowers in extra-axillary few-flowered cymes, sometimes reduced to a single flower; peduncles short; pedicels short, curved, stellately hairy.

Calyx

Calyx 5 lobed, nearly 1.3 cm long, densely hairy and prickly; tube short, globose, lobes 11 mm long, linear-lanceolate, acute, prickly outside, enlarged in fruit.

Corolla

Corolla purple, 2 cm long, lobes deltoid, acute, hairy outside, rotate, tube short, limb plicate, 5-lobed.

Androecium

Stamens 5, in the corolla-throat; filaments short, 1.5 mm long, glabrous; anthers 8 mm long, oblong-lanceolate, opening by small pores; anthers connivent in a short cone.

Gynoecium

Ovary 2-celled, ovoid, glabrous; style columnar, glabrous; stigma small.

Fruit

Berry small, 1.3–2 cm diam., globose, yellow, or white with green veins surrounded by the enlarged calyx.

Seeds

Seeds numerous, usually discoid; 2.5 mm diam., glabrous; embryo peripheric.

Species and Varieties

At present there is no named or certified varieties under this crop under cultivation.

Plant Parts Used

Root, whole plant, fruit, seed.

Chemical Component

The plant produces 10.8 per cent ash (soluble 7.6 per cent) consisting mainly of potassium nitrate, carbonate and sulphate. It also contains 1.6 per cent total sugars of which reducing sugars as glucose is 0.3 per cent, fatty acid and resinous substances. The fruit contains solasonine (3.5 per cent) a glycoalkaloid compound. Seeds contain a greenish yellow oil (19.3 per cent) with a characteristic odour. The component fatty acids of the oil are: oleic acid (45.4 per cent), linoleic acid (38.2 per cent), palmitic acid (5.7 per cent), stearic acid (10.3 per cent) and arachidic acid (0.4 per cent). The unsaponifiable matter contains two sterols, one of which is carpesterol.

Cultivation Procedure

Soil

The plant is very hardy and thrives in different kinds of soil including dry, stony, shallow or deep ones. It grows as a weed throughout dry parts of India. Deep sandy loam to loam soils of medium fertility are however, preferred for its large scale cultivation.

Climatic Requirements

The distribution of the plant makes it apparent that there is no specificity in its climatic requirements. It comes up well in tropical and subtropical areas. However, the growth in tropical areas is better than in the subtropical areas, where its growth is slow due to low temperature in winter. The crop prefers warm, dry conditions all round the year and remains for 150–180 days in field. Where rainfall is high and well-distributed, it can be grown as a rainfed crop. It can be successfully grown up to an elevation of 1,300 m above sea-level.

Method of Propagation

Propagation is mostly done from seeds. Fresh seeds collected from healthy ripe fruits are sown in well-prepared, raised nursery beds in April–May by broadcasting in rows at 8–10 cm apart and at about 1.5 cm depth. They are then covered with a light soil and leaf-mould mixture at 1: 1 ratio and watered to keep the bed moist. For one hectare area of land, 500 g of seeds are sufficient. The seeds germinate within 15–20 days after sowing. The 25–30 days-old seedlings, which are 12–15 cm tall, are ready for transplanting.

Land Preparation

The land is repeatedly ploughed and brought to a fine tilth and weeds, stubbles and pebbles are to be removed. The field is divided into plots of convenient size and the soil is mixed with recommended dose of manures. About 20–25 tones of FYM is required for an hectare area of land. Groundnut cake, bone-meal, rapeseed cake and vermicompost are also beneficial for better growth of the plants. To remove mites and nematods from the field, prior application of neem cake is recommended at the doses of 7–12 kg/ha.

Planting

The seedlings are transplanted in rows at 60 cm apart in well-prepared field. A plant population of 40,000 plants/ha is optimum.

Manuring

In low fertile soil, 20–25 tonns of FYM/ha is recommended but in moderately fertile condition, the dose may be reduced at 15–18 tonns/ha. If irrigation facilities are available, it is recommended to green manure the field with leguminous crops. The seeds of the green manure crop may be treated with the bacterial inoculants before sowing so as to increase the development of root nodules which absorb atmospheric nitrogen and fix it into the soil.

Irrigation

The plants are drought resistant and do not require much water but irrigations in summer is helpful.

Intercultural Measures

The crop responds well by 2–3 periodic hoeing and weeding at interval of 20 or 30 days. Mulching with rice straw or cut-grass is recommended to minimise weed growth.

At early flowering stage, the top 2 cm portions of the plant are removed to promote vegetative growth and enhance the alkaloid content. At early flowering stage, the top 2 cm portions of the plant are removed to promote vegetative growth and enhance the alkaloid content.

Intercropping

The plants may be grown as an itnercrop with any shrub or tree.

Crop Protection Measures

The plants are practically free from the attack of any serious pest or disease.

Harvesting

Roots

The Crop is ready to harvest after 12 months of sowing. About 150 days after sowing or transplanting, the periwinkle roots penetrate the soil up to 15-25 cm and then produce lateral rootlets. The plants are cut about 7.5 cm above the ground level and dried for the stems, leaves & seeds. The field is then copiously irrigated and when the field reaches the proper condition for digging, it is ploughed and the roots are collected and washed.

Leaves, Stems and Seeds

Two leaf strippings are done, the first after 6 months and second after 9 months of sowing. Third leaf stripping is also obtained when whole plant is harvested.

The leaves and stems are collected separately. The aerial part of the plant between 7.5 cm and about 25 cm above the ground level is taken as the stem crop after whole plant is harvested.

In the case of seed, they are collected after the total plant is harvested and dried in the shade. The seed pod dehisce and release the seeds with a light threshing. To collect the seeds for breeding purpose, it is advisable to collect them from mature pods two or three months before the harvest of the crop.

Post-harvest Processing

Root

The roots are washed properly, then cut into pieces of 15–25 cm length and dried.

Stem

The basal stems upto 10 cm long, are separated from roots and cut into pieces and dried.

Leaves

The harvested leaves are dried in shade and stored in gunny bags.

Seeds

Seeds are collected by a light threshing to the dried seed pods of harvested dried plants.

Yield

The total biomass yield goes to 1.0–1.2 tonns/ha under rainfed condition and may increase to 1.7–2.0 tonns for an irrigated crop.

Medicinal Properties

The root is pungent, bitter, appetiser, laxative, stomachic, anthelmintic and useful in bronchitis, asthma, fever, ozaena, strangury, lumbago, pains, piles, thirst, urinary concertions and diseases of the heart. The fruit is bitter, digestible, improves appetite and is helpful in diseases of the heart, prúritus, asthma, fever, intestinal worm etc.

The root is known to be an aphrodisiac and the leaves are used in piles. It is valued in cough, asthma, catarrhal fever and pain in the chest. A decoction of the root is given with the addition of long paper and honey, in cough and catarrh and with rock salt and assafoetide in spasmodic cough.

The roots mixed up with wine are given to check vomitting. The juice of the berries is also used in sore throat.

The stems, flowers and fruits are carminative and are prescribed in those forms of the burning of the feet (*Ignipeditis*) which are attended with a vesicular, watery eruption. Fumigation with the vapour of the burning seeds of this plant are in high repute in the cure of toothache. It acts as a powerful sialogogue, and by this means probably relief is obtained.

Fruits are esteemed for curries. Seeds also are eaten. The plant is known to have anti-hypertensic effective and is beneficial in bronchial asthma for its role in reducing the level of histamine.

Appendices

Appendix I

Glossary of Some Selected Pharmaceutical Terms

Abscess: A localised collection of pus anywhere in the body, surrounded and walled off by damaged and inflamed tissues.

Acidemia: A condition of abnormally high blood acidity.

Acidity: Sourness, a sign of indigestion (under digestive disorders due to excessive secretion of HCl)

Acne vulgaris: Skin eruptions on inflammatory base, occurs usually during puberty and adolescence.

Acrosclerosis: Skin disease thought to be a type of generalized "Scleroderma".

Acute rheumatism (*Rheumatic fever*): Disease affecting mainly children and young adults that arises as a delayed complication of infection of the upper respiratory tract with hemolytic streptococci.

Adenitis: Inflammation of gland or group of glands.

Adenosis: Any disease of a gland, especially of a lymph node.

Alastrim: A mild form of smallpox, causing only a sparse rash and low-grade fever.

Alkalemia: A condition of abnormally high blood alkalinity.

Allergen: Any antigen that causes allergy in a hypersensitive person.

Alopecia (*Baldness*): Absence of hair from areas where it normally grows.

Amebiasis (*Amebic dysentery*): An infection caused by the protozoan *Entamoeba histolytica* resuting ulceration of the intestinal tract causing severe diarrhoea with blood and mucus.

Amenorrhoea: Abnormal suppression or absence of menstrual period.

Amnesia: Total or partial loss of memory following physical injury, disease, drugs or psychological trauma.

Anaemia: A condition caused by qualitative and quantitative reduction of red blood corpuscles and or haemoglobin.

Analgesic: A drug that relieves pain.

Anesthetic: An agent that reduces or abolishes sensation, affecting either the whole body (general anesthetic) or a particular region (local anesthetic)

Angina: A sense of suffocation or suffocating pain.

Anasarca: Oedema in subcutaneous tissues all over the body.

Angitis: A patchy inflammation of the walls of small blood vessels.

Anorexia: Loss of appetite.

Antacid: A drug that neutralizes the hydrochloric acid secreted in the digestive juices of the stomach.

Anthelmintic: A drug or chemcial agent that destroy parasitic worms or remove them from the body.

Antiallergic: Agent that counters allergic reactions.

Antibacterial: An agent capable of reducing or stopping the action and proliferation of bacteria.

Anticonvulsant: A drug that prevents or reduces the severity of convulsions in various types of epilepsy.

Antidepressant: A drug that alleviates the symptoms of depression.

Antiemetic: Agent which prevents or lessens tendency to vomit.

Antifertility: A drug that inhibits formation of ova or sperm or interferes with the process of fertilisation.

Antihelmintic: A drug that acts against helminths.

Antilithic: Which prevents the formation of calculii or promotes their dissolution.

Antipuritic: An agent that relieves itching.

Antipyretic: Agent that reduces body temperature, i. e. fever.

Antiscorbutic: A drug that cures scurvy.

Antiseptic: Agent that arrests development or reproduction of bacteria and other microorganisms.

Antispasmodic: Allays, relaxes or control spasms.

Antiviral: Agent to treat or stop viral infection.

Aperient: Mild laxative.

Aphthae: A boil in mucus membrane in mouth.

Apoplexy: A general term for cerebral haemorrhage, thrombosis, vasospasm.

Appendicitis: Inflammation of the vermiform appendix of the ceacum.

Appetiser: An agent which stimulates appetite.

Aromatic: Substance having pleasant smell or flavour.

Arthritis: Inflammation of joint(s)

Ascaris: A genus of parasitic worms infecting small intestine.

Ascites: Abnormal accumulation of serous fluid in peritoneal cavity of abdomen.

Asthma: A lung disease characterised by wheezing, difficult breathing and feeling of suffocation.

Astringent: An agent which contracts tissues and checks secretions.

Atrophy: Wasting away of a normally developed organ or tissue due to degeneration of cells.

Beri-beri: A nutritional disorder due to deficiency of vitamin B_1.

Biliousness: Containing bile with fluid.

Bite: Cut into or nip with the teeth by dog, jackle and other wild animals.

Blister: Vesicle on skin filled with serum caused by friction, burning etc.

Blood pressure: The pressure caused on the walls of blood vessels due to the flow and pumping of the blood by heart.

Blood purifier: Agents believed to remove impurities from or deficiencies of blood.

Blood sugar: Sugar in blood, if the level of its concentration goes beyond certain limit, causes a disease called diabetes.

Boil: A tender inflammed area of the skin containing pus.

Bone fracture: Breaking of a bone.

Bronchitis: Inflammation of bronchi.

Burn: Tissue damaged, caused by such agents as heat, chemicals, electricity, sunlight or nuclear radiation.

Burning sensation inside body: Includes feeling hot inside the body or in palms, soles etc.

Calculus: Deposit of solid matter, like salts, in any part of the body, such as kidney, gall bladder.

Cancer: A malignant new growth or tumour in any part of the body.

Carbuncle: An extensive boil which discharges pus from many points.

Cardiac complaint: Ailments relating to heart.

Caries: Decay or rottenness or ulceration of bone, it is related to teeth.

Carminative: The medicine which cures flatulence, promotes expulsion from or reduces formation of gas in stomach.

Cataract: Opacity or clouding of lens of eye causing partial blindness.

Catarrh: Inflammation of mucous membranes.

Cerebral affections: Ailment of cerebral region.

Chancre: Sore caused by syphilis.

Chicken pox: A contagious disease resulting in eruption of papules.

Chilblain: Localised inflammation of skin in cold weather.

Cholera: An acute infectious disease caused by *Vibrio cholerae* resulting in diarrhoea, vomiting, cramps and suppression of urine.

Cirrhosis: Diminution and deformity of liver due to necrosis followed by fibrosis.

Cold: Exposure to cold or sudden change of temperature causing inflammed state of mucous membrane with hoarseness of voice, running nose, sore throat, etc.

Colic: Severe gripping pains to contraction of muscles in walls of intestines.

Conjuctivitis: Inflammation of conjuctiva.

Constipation: Costiveness, condition of bowels when defection of faeces is irregular of difficult.

Consumption: Wasting of tissues, tuberculosis.

Contraceptive: A drug or device to prevent unwanted pregnancy.

Contusion: Injury to tissues by blow without causing break in skin.

Convulsion: Violent irregular motion of limb or body due to involuntary contraction of muscles.

Cooling: Reducing temperature or thirst.

Corn: Horny induration of cuticle with hard centre and root, often penetrating deep into subjacent tissue, caused by pressure of shoe or feet.

Cough: A violent effort of the lungs to throw off injurious matter accompanied by harsh sound from throat.

Cramp: Prolonged painful involuntary contraction of muscles.

Cut: Breaking of skin due to external means.

Dandruff: Scurf; dead skin in small scales among hairs.

Dehydration: Loss or deficiency of water in body tissues.

Delirium: Derangement of mental functions accompanied with incoherent speech.

Demulcent: Substance to soothen mucous membrane and releives irritation.

Dermatitis: Inflammation of skin causing discomforts.

Diabetes: A metabolic disorder resulting in elevated blood glucose.

Diaphoretic: Drug or treatment causing sweating or perspiration.

Diarrhoea: A common symptom of gastrointestinal diseases resulting in excessive looseness of bowels accompanied with frequent discharge of watery stool.

Diphtheria: An acute infectious disease with inflammation of mucous membrane of throat in which air passages become covered and impeded by leathery membrane.

Disinfectant: A substance which destroys harmful germs, cleans infections.

Diuretic: An agent that induces passing of urine.

Dropsy: See Oedema

Dysentery: A disease caused by bacteria or protozoa causing infection in the intestinal tract with severe diarrhoea with blood and mucus.

Dyspepsia: Indigestion.

Dysuria: Difficult or painful urination.

Ecbolic: An agent which hastens delivery or produces abortion.

Eczema: Acute or chronic noncontagious inflammation of skin often accompanied by itching.

Elephantiasis: Enlargement of cutaneous and subcutaneous tissues caused by obstruction of lymphatics–the affected part resembles elepahant's hide.

Emetic: Causes or produces vomiting.

Emmenagogue: A substance which stimulates normal menstrual function.

Emollient: A substance applied externally to soften and soothes the skin.

Epilepsy: A nervous disorder causing temporary loss of consciousness with or without convulsions.

Eruption: Any lesion that appears at the surface of the skin and is characterized by its prominence and redness.

Erysipelas: Local febrile disease, producing deep red colour on skin and subcutaneous tissue.

Expectorant: Which promotes ejection of phlegm, etc., from chest or lungs by regulating bronchial secretions.

Epistaxis: Nasal haemorrhage.

Fertility: Capability to conceive or cause conception.

Fever: Abnormal raise of body temperature and quickening of pulse.

Filaria: A term for a group of worms of Filarioidea family.

Fistula: An abnormal communication between two hollow organs or between two layers of a organ and the exterior.

Fit: A sudden attack by convulsions.

Flatulence: Excessive gas in stomach and intestine.

Galactahogue: A substance which induces or stimulates secretion of milk.

Gangrene: Necrosis, usually with loss of vitality or decomposition in some part of the body.

Germicide: Agent that destroy germ.

Giddiness: Dizziness, feeling of things circling round the person causing instability.

Goiter: Morbid enlargement of thyroid gland, often showing as large pendulous swelling in neck.

Gonorrhoea: A veneral disease, inflammatory discharge of mucus from urethra or vagina.

Gout: A constitutional condition of uric acid metabolism, resulting painful inflammation of smaller joints.

Guinea worm: A thread-like tropical parasitic nematode.

Haematoma: Collection of blood at some part of body due to trauma.

Haematuria: Presence of red blood corpuscles in urine.

Haemoptysis: Spitting of blood from bronchi, larynx, lungs or trachea.

Haemorrhage: Discharge of blood from blood vessels.

Haemorrhoids: Piles with painful swelling at the anus.

Haemostat: Agent that arrests bleeding.

Hallucinogenic: A drug or substance that produces hallucinations, imaginary things apparently seen or heard.

Headache: Pain in head.

Hemicrania: Severe pain affecting one side of head, usually migraine.

Hemiplegia: Paralysis of one side of body.

Hepatitis: Inflammation of liver.

Hernia: Abnormal protrusion of an organ through its containing wall, usually associated with abdominal cavity.

Hydrocele: Pathological accumulation of serum fluid in body cavity, especially in the testes.

Hydrophobia: Dread of water with convulsions, generally caused by rabies.

Hypertension: High blood pressure.

Hypnotic: Sleep inducing.

Hypoglycemic: Low level of sugar in blood.

Hypotensive: Agent to reduce blood pressure.

Hysteria: A functional disturbance of nervous system of psychoneurotic origin, especially in women, characterised by convulsions, and usually attended with disturbance of intellectual faculty.

Impotence: Inability to engage in sexual intercourse.

Indigestion: Digestive disorder.

Inflammation: Morbid process affecting any part or organ of the body with swelling, heat, pain and redness.

Infertility: Incapability to conceive or cause conception.

Influenza: A severe epidemic febrile disease with rapid prostration; severe catarrh and weakening fever.

Injury: Contusion, cut, wound, bruise caused by external hit.

Insomnia: Sleeplessness.

Intoxication: State of being drunk, high excitement beyond self control.

Itch: Irritation in skin.

Jaundice: Morbid state caused by obstruction of bile, and marked by yellowness of skin, loss of appetite.

Joint disease: Variety of painful diseases causing swelling, immobility and even deformation of joints.

Labour: Pains of child birth.

Lactagogue: Which promotes secretion and flow of milk.

Lactation problems: Disfunctions of mammary glands.

Laxative: Medicine tending to loosen bowels.

Leprosy: Chronic contagious diseases due to infection with *Lepra bacillus*, varying in manifestation as the skin, nerve or other tissues are affected.

Leucoderma: A skin condition characterised by defective whitish pigmentation, vitiligo.

Leucorrhoea: A white or yellowish mucopurulent discharge from vagina.

Lithotriptic: The agent which causes dissolution of a calculus.

Loose motion: Watery motion.

Lumbago: Rheumatic affection in loins.

Malaria: An acute or chronic disease, usually accompanied with intermittent and remittent fever, caused by protozoa (*Plasmodium* sp.) and transmitted by female Anopheles mosquito.

Masticatory: Substance chewed for increased salivation.

Measles: An acute infectious disease, caused by virus infection, and marked by red pustules.

Melancholia: A disease of mind marked by sadness, depression and illgrounded fears.

Menorrhagia: Diseases associated with menstruation including premenstrual tension.

Migraine: A recurring and very painful headache on one side of the head, often accompanied by giddiness, vomiting.

Miscarriage: Premature involuntary expulsion of foetus.

Mumps: Virus infection which caused acute inflammation of parotid and salivary glands.

Narcotic: Substance which tends to induce drowsiness, sleep, stupor, even paralysis of nervous system.

Nausea: Sensation of sickness of stomach, which may cause vomiting.

Nephritis: Inflammation of kidney(s)

Neuralgia: Sudden severe pain radiating along the course of a nerve.

Neurosis: A disease of nerve(s)

Night blindness: Inability to see in dim light.

Oedema: Flow of excessive clear fluid from blood into other tissue(s)

Oxytocic: Any drug that hastens child birth.

Pain: Distress of body, like bodyache, headache, muscular pain, etc.

Paralysis: Loss of power of motion.

Parturition: The act of child birth.

Piles: Enlarged or dilated blood vessels; disease marked by elongation of ano-rectal vain.

Pimple: Small, inflammed swelling and outgrowth on skin.

Pleurisy: Inflammation of the pleura membrane enveloping lung, usually caused by chill and marked by pain in chest or side, fever, etc.

Pneumonia: Inflammation or congestion in lungs.

Poison: Toxic substance.

Polyuria: Excessive micturition.

Postnatal: After child birth.

Prenatal: Before child birth, generally related to obstratical or other problems related to pregnancy.

Prickly heat: Heat rash, irritation of the skin caused by heat.

Pruritus: Itching.

Psoriasis: A auto-immuno inflammatory skin disease with reddish patches covered with white scales.

Purgative: The agent which causes evacuation of bowels.

Pyorrhoea: A purulent discharge with pus.

Rabies: Canine madness, an infectious viral disease caused in man by bite of infected dogs and some other canine animals.

Refrigerant: Having cooling properties on surface of body.

Rheumatism: A general term; refractory disease of muscle, tendon, joint, bone, nerve, resulting in discomfort and disability.

Rhinitis: Inflammation of the mucous membrane of the nose.

Rickets: A vitamin D deficiency disease of the young, affecting the development of bone.

Ringworm: A common parasitic fungus contagious desease on skin.

Rubefacient: An agent that stimulates skin to redness and increase flow of blood in that part.

Scabies: A contagious parasitic disease of skin causing itching.

Scorpion-sting: Sting by scorpion, usually causing severe irritation and pain.

Scrofula: Tuberculosis of the lymphatic glands, morbid constitutional condition with glandular swellings and tendency to consumption.

Scurvy: A nutritional disorder with swollen gums, livid spots, etc., caused by deficiency of ascorbic acid.

Sedative: Drug which has a calming effect, to releaving anxiety and tention.

Sinus: From sinusitis, the inflammation of sinus.

Skin diseases: Diseases like scabies, ringworm, eczema, fissures and emollients.

Small pox: A severe and fatal disease with eruptions on skin and fever due to pox virus infection.

Snake bite: Cut by snake.

Soporific: Agent that produces sleep.

Sore: A general term for variety of morbidly tender tisues, boils and wounds.

Spasmolytic: A drug that prevents spasm.

Spermatorrhoea: Involuntary semen-dischage.

Spleen complains: Disorder in spleen function.

Splenomegaly: Enlargement of spleen.

Sprain: The wrench or twist of a ligament or muscle or a joint causing pain and swelling.

Sprue: Intestinal malabsorption with steatorrhoea.

Steriliser: An agent that destroys unwanted bacteria or other pathogens.

Sterility: Incapability to conceive or cause conception.

Stimulant: An agent that increases functional activity of an organ.

Stomachache: Pain or unspecified disorder in stomach.

Stupor: A condition of near unconsciousness, with apparent mental inactivity and reduced ability to respond to stimulation.

Stye: A small inflammated gland on base of eyelash.

Sudorific: That which causes perspiration.

Sun stroke: Exposure to excessive heat, raised body temperature, absence of perspiration and eventual loss of consciousness due to failure of exhaustion of the temperature regulating mechanism.

Syphilis: A contagious venereal disease caused by *Treponema pallidium*.

Tetanus: An infectious disease caused by bacillus *Clostridium tetani* and marked by spasm of many or all muscles of voluntary motion.

Tonic: A drug that invigorates or improves normal tone of the body and produce a feeling of wellbeing.

Tonsilitis: Inflammation of the tonsil(s)

Tuberculosis: An infectious disease caused by *Mycobacterium tuberculosis*.

Tumour: Generally an abnormal growth of tissue.

Typhoid: Infectious desease caused by waterborne bacteria, *Salmonella typhi*.

Ulcer: An open sore on external or internal surface of body, that fails to heal.

Unconsciousness: The state of absence of consciousness.

Urethritis: Inflammation of urethra.

Urinary complaints: Disorder in urinary system, *e.g.*, blood in urine, dysuria, night wetting, haematuria, urethritis. etc.

Uterine disorders: Irregularity in the normal function of the uterus.

Venereal diseases: Diseases communicated by sexual intercourse, *viz.* gonorrhoea, syphilis etc.

Virtigo: Giddiness, dizziness in which patient fells that he himself or his surrounding objects are whirling.

Vesicant: Any agent that causes blisters.

Veternary: Ailments of domestic animals and birds.

Vomiting: Throwing up the contents of the stomach by mouth.

Weakness: A feeling of loss or reduction in normal strength of body.

Whooping cough: An infectious diseases found among children caused by *Hemophilus pertussis.*

Worms: A variety of limbless or apparently limbless creeping creatures which are parasites on human body, mainly in the intestinal tract.

Wound: Incision in soft tissues of skin caused by external injury.

Appendix II

Glossary of Some Selected Botanical Terms

Accrescent: Enlarging with age.

Achene: Small, dry, hard, one-chambered, one-seeded fruit.

Acicular: Needle-shaped.

Actinomorphic: Flower having radial symmetry.

Acuminate: Suddenly tapering to a sharp point.

Acyclic: Arranged in spirals and not in whorls.

Adnate: Adherent.

Albuminous: Provided with albumen or endosperm.

Alternate: One leaf at a node, and leaves are so arranged that a line connecting the consecutive leafbases will take a spiral course on the stem.

Amplexicaul: Leafbase embracing the stem completely.

Androgynous: Bearing staminate and carpellat flowers in the same inflorescence.

Annual: Plants which complete their life-cycle withing a year.

Anther: Pollen containing part of a stamen.

Apetalous: Absence of petals.

Aril: A small appendage from or around the hilum of a seed.

Articulate: Jointed.

Asepalous: Without sepals.

Attenuate: Drawn out into a long, slender extension.

Auricle: An earshaped appendaged, normally form the top of the leafsheath in grasses.

Awn: Bristle-like appendage.

Axil: The angular space between stem and leafstalk.

Baccate: Having the nature of berry, pulpy or fleshy.

Basifixed: Filament attached to the base of the anther.

Balausta: Fruit with firm rind, berried within and crowned with lobes of adnate calyx.

Barbed: Equipped with retrorse projections.

Barbellate: Finely barbed.

Berry: Fleshy, indehiscent, few to many seeded fruit derived from a gynoecium of fused carples.

Bicarpellary: Pistil with two carples.

Biennial: The plant which completes it life-cycle in two years.

Bifid: Two-celft.

Bifoliate: A comound leaf having two leaflets.

Bilabiate: Two-lipped, referring especially to zygomorphic corolla.

Bilocular: Two-chambered.

Bipinnate: Twice pinnate, rachis (modified midrib) producing secondary axes which bear leaflets.

Bisexual: When androecium and gynoecium present in the same flower.

Blade: Expanded flat part of a leaf.

Bract: Modified leaf at the base of a flower.

Bractlet: Bract borne on a secondary axis.

Bracteate: Bract present.

Brateole: Secondary bract.

Bracteolate: With barcteoles.

Bulb: Modified underground stem, most of the leaves of which are thickened at the base with stored reserve food.

Bulbil: Modified axillary vegegative or floral bud.

Caducous: Falling off early.

Calyculus: Simulated calyx composed of bracts and bracteoles but not of sepals.

Calyx: The outermost, generally green, floral envelope.

Caylx tube: The tube formated by calyx.

Campanulate: Bell-shaped.

Campylotropous: The ovule is so bent as to bring the hilum, micropyle and chalaza close together.

Canescent: Bearing greyish hairs.

Capitate: Headlike.

Capsule: Dry, dehiscent fruit, developed from a compound gynoecium (constituted of two or more carpels), splitting along two or more lines of suture.

Carcerules: Dry schizocarpic fruit, developed from a bicarpellary ovary, and ultimately breaking into four nutlets.

Cardiopetalous: With heart-shaped petals.

Carpel: The ovuliferous organ of the flower; often regarded as a single, modified megaspore-bearing leaf.

Caryopsis: Small, dry, indehiscent, one seeded fruit in which the seedcoat is adherent to the wall of fruit.

Caryophyllaceous: Five petals with comparatively long claws, and limbs placed at right anlges to the claws.

Catkin: An elongate spike with compartively soft axis, which failing to bear the weight of flowers, bends down.

Caudate: Bearing a tail-like appendage–normally the term is applied to leaf-apex.

Caudex: The type of stem found in palms.

Cauline: Borne of the stem only.

Centric: A leaf which is more or less cylindrical.

Circinate: A prefoliate state of a leaf where the leaf remains coiled or rolled from apex to base like the tail of a dog.

Cirrhose: A slender coiled apex.

Cladode: Cylindrical or flattened green branch of one internode or of limited growth.

Clavate: Club-shaped, gradually thickened upwards.

Claw: Narrow basal part of a petal.

Cleistogamous: Flowers which remain closed to ensure self-pollination.

Climber: A plant which attaches itself to a nearby support by means of some special device for growing upwards.

Coccus: Spherial structure; a part of a schizocarpic fruit.

Cochleate: Shaped like a spiral shell.

Coherent: Fused or united with the organs of same kind.

Cohesion: The phenomenon of union of similar organs, *viz.*, union of sepals or petals or stamens.

Coleoptile: The sheath surrounding the young stem of grasses.

Coleorhiz: The sheath surrounding the young root of grasses.

Collateral: Placed side by side.

Comose: Leaf surface bearing a tuft or tufts of hairs.

Complete: A flower having all four sets of floral organs.

Complicate: When the leafblade is folded upon itself.

Conduplicate: The pattern of a leaf in which the blade is folded lengthwise with the upper surface within.

Confluent: Blended into one.

Conical: Cone-like–broad at the base and gradually tapering towards the apex.

Connate: When the bases of some organs appear to have fused.

Connective: The part of a stamen which joins two anther sacs.

Connivent: Coming close together or touching similar organs but not united.

Convolute: Longitudinally rolled up from one margin to other like the rolling up of a sheet of paper.

Cordate: Heart-shaped with a basal notch.

Coriaceous: Leathry.

Corm: A stout, solid, fleshy, underground stem growing in the vertical direction.

Corneous: Horny texture.

Corolla: Second outer whorl of a flower, consists of a number of petals.

Corona: Collar-like or tubular appendage of corolla, forming more or less a crown like structure.

Corrugate: Wrinkled or folded having prominent ridges.

Corymb: A type of racemose inflorescence where the main axis is comparatively short, and the lower flowers have longer stalks or pedicels than upper ones so that all the flowers are brought to more or less same level.

Corymbose: Corymb-like.

Cotyloid: A concave receptacle, sometimes to the extent of surrounding the carpels.

Creeper: A trailing shoot that produces roots from nodes, almost throughout its length.

Cremocarp: Dry, dehiscent, two seeded fruit, each half a mericarp, borne on a thread-like carpophore.

Crenate: Shallowly rounded or obtusely toothed margin.

Crenulate: Finely crenate.

Crispate: An extreme form of undulate.

Cruciform: Cross-shaped.

Crustaceous: Hard and brittle texture.

Culm: Jointed stem with solid nodes and hollow internodes.

Cuneate: Wedge-shaped with broad apical end.

Cupule: A small cup-shaped structure formed usually by fusion of bracts together.

Cuspidate: Ending in a sharp rigid point.

Cyamium: A kind of follicle.

Cyathium: A special type of inflorescence, where the involucre is cup-shaped; it encloses a single reduced female flower, surrounded by a number of reduced male flowers.

Cyme: A determinate inflorescence, where the apical flower opens first.

Cynarrhodion: A fleshy hollow fruit enclosing achenes.

Cypsela: An achene developed from an inferior ovary and invested by an adnate calyx.

Deciduous: Falling off soon after maturity; not persistent.

Decompound: Applied to a compound leaf when the leaf is more than thrice pinnate.

Decumbent: Reclining or growing flat along the ground, but with the tip ascending.

Decurrent: The leafblade appearing to extend down the sides of the stem and adnate to the stem.

Decussate: Applied to leaves which occur in pairs alternately at right angles at adjacent nodes.

Deltoid: Like a delta; trinagular.

Dentate: Usually applied to leaf margins, where the margin bears sharp teeth directed outwards at right angles to the margin.

Denticulate: Minutely toothed leaf margin.

Diadelphous: Name of stamens, when the stamens are grouped into two bundles.

Diandrous: Applied to flowers which bear two stamens only.

Dichasium: A type of cymose inflorescence, where the main axis end in a flower and at the same time it produces two leteral younger flowers; the process is repeated by each set of branches.

Dichlamydous: Applied to flowers having both whorls of perianth, *i.e.* calyx and corolla.

Dichogamous: Name of flowers in which stamens and carples mature at different times.

Dichotomy: A pattern of branching where the axes divides into two equal halves.

Diclinous: Applied to plants/flowers when androecium and gynoecium are borne on separate flowers.

Didynamous: Androecium having four stamens in two pairs of different lengths.

Diffuse: Plants having stem spread over the ground.

Digitate: A palmately compound leaf in which the petiole bears terminally a number of leaflets which appear to be radiating from a common point like fingers from the palm.

Dimerous: Applied to flowers when each whorl consists of two units.

Dimorphic: Those have two forms.

Dioecius: Plants having male and female flowers borne on different individuals.

Disk: Outgrowth of the receptacle, may be epignous or hypogynous.

Dissected: Deeply divided or cut into many slender segments.

Disk florets: Tubular flowers in the centre of a capitulum.

Divided: Separated very near the base.

Dorsifixed: Filament attached to the back of anther.

Dorsiventral: Flattened structure with distinct dorsal (upper) and ventral (lower) surfaces.

Drupaceous: Resembling a drupe.

Drup: The fleshy, one-seeded, indehiscent fruit with the seed enclosed in a stony endocarp, while the mesocarp remains thick and fleshy and the epicarp thin.

Echinate: Beset with prickles.

Emerginate: With a shallow notch at the apex.

Emergence: An outgrowth developing from superficial layers.

Endocarp: Intermost zone of pericarp.

Endosperm: The food-storage tissue of grain, which normally stores proteinaceous food; this nutritive tissue normally nourishes the embryo in seed plants.

Ensiform: Sword-shaped.

Entire: Even and smooth without any marginal serrations.

Entomophillous: Insect loving; the term usually refers to insect pollinated flowers.

Epicalyx: The whorl of sepaloid green structures just outside and below the calyx.

Epicarp: The outermost zone of pericarp.

Epigynous: Situated upon or on top of the ovary.

Epipetalous: Borne upon petals, nomally referred to the stamens occuring on petals.

Epiphyte: A plant growing upon another plant but using it as support only and not drawing nutrition from the latter.

Equitant: Conduplicate leaves standing face to face and one completely overlapping the other by both the margins.

Erect: A rigid, firm stem itself in an upright position.

Erose: Irregularly toothed.

Exasperate: Rough with hard projecting points.

Extipulate: Stipules are absent.

Extra-axillary: Situated outside the axil.

Extrorse: Facing outwards.

Falcate: Sickle-shaped or scythe-shaped.

False fruit: A fruit not developed from a fertilized ovary, but from some other part(s) of a flower.

Farinaceous: Either containing starch or starch-like materials in nature.

Fasciculated: Clustered or bundled, normally applied to root.

Filiform: Like a filament or thread.

Fimbriae: Fringed along the edge.

Fistular: Stem or leaf having a hollow interior throughout its length.

Flabellate: Fan-shaped.

Flaccid: Flabby, withered and limp.

Flocoose: With tufts of silky or woolly hairs that rub off easily.

Floret: Reduced flower.

Foliaceous: Leaf-like.

Follicle: A dry one-chambered fruit developed from single carpel, and splits along one suture only.

Free-lateral: Free and situated on sides–usually applied in respect of stipules.

Fruticose: Shrub-like.

Fugacious: Withers as soon as formed.

Funicle or Funiculus: The slender stalk of the ovule, by which it remains attached to the placenta.

Fusiform: Spindle-shaped, narrowed both ways from a swollen middle.

Gamopetalous: With united petals.

Gamophyllous: Perianth with united segments.

Gamosepalous: With united sepals.

Gibbous: Tubula; structure having the base or one side slightly dilated to a pouch; this term is usually applied to corolla.

Glabrous: A structure having its surface smooth and free hairs or outgrowths of any kind.

Glandular: Possessing gland(s)

Gland-dotted: When glands are scattered like dots on a surface.

Glaucous: The surface is covered by a waxy coating causing a shiny bluish or whitish tinge.

Globose: Spherical like a globe.

Glochidium: A barbed bristle.

Glochidate: Equipped with barbed bristles.

Glumaceous: Glume-like.

Glume: Chaff-like scaly bracts, usually found in the grasses and similar plants.

Glutinous: Covered with a sticky exudation.

Gregarious: Growing in clusters.

Gynandrophore: The internode of the thalamus between corolla and androecium.

Gynandrous: Usually refers to the stamens which are adnate to carples as a whole or by their anthers only.

Gynobasic: Applied to the style which arises from the depressed centre of a syncarpous ovary, actually the style adheres by its base to the prolongation of the torus upwards between the carpels.

Gynophore: The elongated internode of the thalamus on which pistil is situated–this looks like a stalk of the pistil.

Gynostegium: A sheath or covering of the gynoecium.

Gynostemium: The column in an orchid flower, formed by adnation of stamens and styles.

Habit: Characteristic appearance of a plant.

Habitat: Natural home of a plant.

Halophyte: A plant which grows in saline substratum.

Hastate: Arrow-shaped leaf with two basal lobes directed outwards.

Head: Capitulum inflorescence.

Helicoid: Coiled like a hellex.

Herb: Small plant with soft stem, may vary from a few millimetres to a metre or so in height.

Herkogamy: The phenomenon of having some sort of barrier between the stamens and the pistil of the same flower.

Hermaphrodite: Bisexual.

Hesperidium: A superior, many-celled, fleshy fruit where the endocarp projects inwards forming distinct chambers, and the mesocarp and epicarp, fused together, form a separable skin, *e.g.* orange and other citrus fruits.

Heteroanthy: The phenomenon of having stamens of different lengths.

Heterogamous: Bearing two kinds of flowers, male and female.

Heteromerous: Refers to a flower where the number of members of different whorls is irregular.

Heteromorphic: Plants bearing two or more different forms of flowers with anthers and stigmas at different levels.

Heterophyllous: The same individual plant bearing different types of leaves.

Heterostyly: When one plant bears some flowers with long styles and others with short styles.

Hilum: The point of attachment of the body of the ovule to its stalk. On a developed seed, it is represented by a scar, indicating the point where the seed breaks from the stalk.

Hirsute: Having moderately stiff separate hairs.

Hispid: Having stiff or bristly hairs.

Hispidulous: Minutely hispid.

Hyaline: Colourless and translucent or transparent.

Hypanthium: The tube of the receptacle upon which the calyx, corolla and stems are borne, perianth tube.

Hypanthodium: It is the typical inflorescence of banyan, fig, etc., where the fleshy receptacle forms a hollow cavity with an apical opening guarded by scales, and the flowers are borne on the inner wall of the cavity.

Hypocotyl: The axis of the embroy lying immediately below the cotyledons.

Imbricate: This is a type of aestivation (mode of arrangement of the sepals or of the petals in a floral bud with respect to the members of the same whorl), where one of the sepals or petals is overlapped on both the margins, and one of them is external, and each of the ramaining one is overlapped on one margin and overlaps the next one on the other margin.

Imparipinnate: A unipinnate leaf with an odd terminal leaflet.

Imperfect flower: A flower missing either stamens or capels, a unisexual flower.

Incised leaf: A leaf with prominently indented margin.

Indehiscent: Applied to fruits which do not open.

Indeterminate: of indefinite growth.

Indigenous: Native to a region.

Infinite: Very great in number, applied to inflorescences indicating indefinite growth.

Inflexed: Leaf with margins turned inwards.

Inflorescence: Arrangement of flowers of a plant in relation to axis and to each other.

Infundibuliform: Funnel-shaped.

Innate: Natural, applied to stamen when the filament is attached to the base of the anther.

Insectivorous: A plant that supplements its nitrogen supply by digesting small insects that become trapped on leaves.

Inserted: Applied to stamens which remain within the flower.

Integument: The envelope of an ovule, which develops to seed-coat in seeds.

Interpetiolar: Between two petioles, usually applied to the stipules.

Introrse: Turned inwards, normally applied to the stamens when the grooved ventral side of anthers faces the centre of the flower.

Involucel: Smaller involucre round the base of each branch of an inflorescence.

Involucre: A whorl of bracts surrounding the base of an inflorescence or several flowers.

Involute: Applied to a leaf in which the two sides are rolled lengthwise over the upper surface towards the midrib.

Irregular: Asymmetrical, applied to flowers or floral parts.

Keel: A prominent dorsal rib or ridge, as in glumes of grasses or in the lower petal of papilionaceous flower or in some carpels.

Kernel: The nucellus of an ovule or of a seed, *i.e.*, the body of seed within the hard shell.

Labiate: Lipped, usually applied to corolla.

Lacerate: Torn.

Laciniate: Cut into deep irregular segments; fringed.

Lacunae: Cavities.

Lanceolate: Lance-shaped, much longer than width, widening above the base and tapering to the apex.

Legume: Dry dehiscent fruit formed from monocarpellary ovary, and splits along both sutures.

Lenticel: Some aerating pores formed in the bark and look like lens-shaped raised spots on the surface of the axis.

Lianas or lianes: Very thick and woody perennial climbers, which twine themselves round tall trees.

Lichen: An extraordinary group of plants; a lichen is a peculiar symbiotic combination of an alga and a fungus.

Ligulate: Furnished with a ligule.

Limb: The broader or expanded part of a gamosepalous celyx or gamopetalous corolla as distinct from a tube or tubular structure.

Linear: Like a line, long and narrow with sides parallel or nearly so.

Lip: One of the fleshy divisions of mouth, the term usually applied to the divisions of a bilabiate calyx or corolla, also applied to that petal in orchids which is larger than the others.

Loculus: Chamber.

Loculicidal: When each loculus splits along the middle of its dorsal suture, the term is applied to some types of dehiscent fruits.

Lodicule: Rudimentary perianth parts, usually found in grass flowers.

Lomentum: A pod constricted or partitioned between the seeds into a number of one-seeded compartments.

Lorate: Star-shaped; ligulate.

Lunate: Half-moon shaped.

Lyrate: Lyer-shaped, applied to pinnatifid leaf with terminal lobe rounded and much larger than the lower ones.

Mericarp: One-seeded indehiscent halves of a cremocarp (fruit of umbellifer family)

Mesocarp: The middle fleshy part of a succulent pericarp.

Mimicry: The phenomenon of copying by the smaller or weaker plants, the general appearance, colour, shape and any particular feature of some dangerous animal.

Monadelphous: Applied to stamens when they are united by their filaments into one bundle.

Monandrous: Flower having one stamen only.

Moniliform: Normally applied to the roots which have some swellings at frequent intervals.

Monocarpellary: With one carpel.

Monogynous: Flower having one carpel or gynoecium.

Monopodial: This term is applied to the nature of branching where the apical bud retians the power of vegetative growth.

Mucronate: Apex (usually of leaf) having an abrupt short sharp point.

Multichasium: A determinate branching (usually inflorescence) having a whorl of many lateral branches.

Muricate: Rough with hard tubercles.

Multiple fruit: A composite fruit that develops from an inflorescence where the flowers are crowded together and often fused with one another.

Nanophanerophyte: Dwarf plants, heights ranging from 25 cm to 2 m, usually found in deserts or in arid zones.

Napiform: Usually applied to roots which are considerably swollen at the upper part, and sharply tapering at the lower part.

Nauseous flower: Flower which emits strong foetid odour during night.

Nectary: A nectar-secreting gland, often associated with petals.

Neuter flower: A flower having no functional stamen or carpel.

Node: The part of the stem which normally bears a leaf and other lateral organs.

Nodulose: Applied to roots having little knob or knot at or near apex.

Nucellus: The tissue in an ovule from which endosperm obtains nutrition.

Nut: A dry, hard-shelled, usually one-seeded indehiscent fruit.

Obcordate: Heart-shaped with the notch at the apex.

Obligate heliophyte: A plant which cannot grow well without being exposed to sunlight.

Oblanceolate: Broader at the distal end and tapering towards the base; often applied to leaf.

Oblique: Unequal sided, resulting in a slanting form.

Oblong: Usually applied to that leaf in which the blade is wide and long with the two margins running straight up.

Obovate: Inversely egg-shaped.

Obturator: A sort plug on the micropyle throgh which the pollen tube may grow; it is usually of placental origin.

Obtuse: When the angle subtended by the margins is more than a right angle, this term is usually applied to leaf apex when the same appears rounded or blunt.

Ochrea: Tubular.

Ochreate: Usually applied to the stipules when they form a hollow tube encircling the stem from node up to certain height of the internode in front of the petiole.

Offset: A short, more or less thickened, horizontal creeping branch of a stem in which the apex turns up and the nodes produce tufts of leaves above and clusters of roots below.

Officinal: Medicinal; sold in apothecaries.

Oosphere: Ovum.

Oospore: Diploid mother cell of the embryo.

Operculum: A lid.

Operculate: Equipped with a lid.

Opposite: Two leaves on opposite sides at a node.

Orbicular: More or less circular.

Ornithophyllus: Flowers pollinated with the aid of birds.

Ornithotropous: Irrate, usually applied to ovules.

Oval: Broadly elliptic.

Ovary: Basal inflated part of a carpel containing ovule(s)

Ovate: Egg-shaped; *i.e.*, broader at the base and narrower at the apex.

Ovule: Megasporanguim (forerunner of seed)

Ovuliferous: Ovule-producing.

Ovum: Haploid egg-cell or oospore.

Oxylophyte: Plant that grows on acid soil.

Palea: The scale-like bracteole found within the lemma or flowering glume of grasses; also the scales on the floral receptacle of many composites.

Paleobotany: That branch of botany which deals with plant fossils.

Palmate: Applied to a compound leaf in which the leaflet arises from a common base at the top of the leafstalk, like the fingers in hand.

Palmati-fid, -partite, -sect: Lobed in the form of a hand, these three terms are applied to indicate the depths of partition between the segments.

Palynology: The science of studying the pollens.

Panicle: Branched inflorescence.

Paniculate: Having panicle.

Papilionaceous: Butterfly-shaped, usually applied to the corolla or some leguminous flowers.

Papilla: Superficial soft protuberance.

Papillose: Clothed with papilla.

Pappose: Equipped with pappus.

Pappus: The modified fine hair-like, bristly or scale-like calyx of each floret of Compositae (Asteraceae); these normally remain attached to the fruits also.

Parachute mechanism: Some fruits and seeds are equipped with some appendages which help the fruits and seeds to float in the air for some time, this mechanism is so named.

Paripinnate: A unipinnate compound leaf bearing even number of leaflets.

Partite: Cleft nearly to the base.

Parietal: Belonging to or borne on wall, usually applied to a type of placentation.

Pectin: A water-soluble chemical, polysachcharied in nature found in the cell-walls and cells of some plants.

Pedate: Palmately lobed leaves where the lobes are arranged like the claw of bird.

Pedicel: The short stalk of a flower brone in an inflorescence.

Pedicellate: Equipped with pedicel.

Peduncle: The main axis of an inflorescence together with lateral axes; when a flower is borne singly, the stalk of the same is also denoted by this term.

Pedunculate: Equipped with a peduncle.

Peltate: Usually referred to such a leaf which is shield-shaped with petiole attached to the centre of the underside.

Pendulous: Hanging like a pendulum.

Pentamerous: Flowers having five (or multiples of five) members in each whorl.

Pentandrous: Flowers having five stamens.

Pepo: One-chambered, many-seeded, fleshy fruit developed from inferior ovary with parietal placentation.

Perennial: Living through many, at least more than two years.

Perfect flower: The flower containing both the essential whorls, *i.e.*, androecium and gynoecium.

Perfoliate: When the base lobes of a leaf fuse together after competely clasping the stem so that it appears that the stem has perforated the leaf, this term is applied.

Perianth: Collective name of the accessory whorls, *i.e.*, calyx and corolla, of a flower.

Pericarp: Wall of the fruit.

Perigynous: Literally means standing around the gynoecium; in some flowers, the thalamus grows upward around the ovary in the form of a cup, carrying on its rim the sepals, petals and stamens, such floral parts and the flower as a whole are called perigynous.

Persistent: Leaves and floral parts which live for long duration; sepals which remain even on the fruits.

Personate: When the two lips of a bilabiate corolla are so placed that the mouth of the corolla remains closed.

Petal: Each constituent of corolla.

Petaloid: Like a petal.

Petiole: The stalk of a leaf.

Phanerogams: Plants with manifest flowers.

Phanerophytes: This term includes trees and shrubs, the plants which are easily visible.

Phylloclade: Green, leaf-like flattened or swollen stem.

Phyllode: A green, flattened petiole which looks like and performs the functions of a lamina.

Phyllotaxy: The various patterns in which the leaves are arranged on the stem.

Pilose: Surface with distinct, soft, long and scattered hairs.

Pinna: A primary division of a pinnately compound leaf.

Pinnate: Feather-like, a compound leaf in which leaflets are arranged in two rows along the common axis.

Pinnatifid: Pinnately parted.

Pinnatisect: Pinnately incised nearly to the rachis.

Pinnule: Secondary pinna.

Pistil: Gynoecium, the whorl consisting of carpels.

Pistillate: Applied to the flower which contains only pistil and not androecium.

Pistillode: A sterile pistil devoid of fertile ovules.

Placentation: Arrangement of placentae (ovule holding tissues) in an ovary.

Pilcate: When a leaf, in bud condition, remains folded longitudinally several times along the prominent ribs.

Plumose: Feathered.

Plumule: The shoot in the emryo.

Pneumathodes: Numerous minute pores of special lenticels found on the exposed parts of breathing roots of halophytes.

Pneumatophores: Negatively geotropic vertical branches bearing pneumathodes.

Pollination: Transference of pollen grains from the anther to the stigma.

Pollinium: A mass of pollen grains adhering together, and shed as a unit.

Polyadelphous: Stamens disposed into several groups by connation of their filaments.

Polyandrous: With indefintie number of stamens.

Polycarpellary: With indefinite number of carpels.

Polygamous: Same plant bearing both unisexual and bisexual flowers.

Polymorphic: Having several forms.

Polypetalous: The corolla in which all the petals remain fre from each other.

Polyphyllous: When all the members of a perianth remain free from each other.

Pome: A type of fleshy fruit which develops from a compound gynoecium with the seeds encased within a cartilaginous wall, and the fruit remains surrounded by fleshy edible thalamus.

Prefoliation: Arrangement of the young leaves in the bud prior to opening.

Prickle: Sharp pointed or curved and unbranched short and superficial outgrowth.

Prop root: Roots developing from the main stem or from the branches, grow downwards and act as pillars supporting the main stem or branches.

Prostrate: Lying flat on the ground.

Protrandous flower: A flower in which the androecium matures before the gynoecium.

Protogynous flower: A flower in which the gynoecium matures earlier than the androecium.

Pseudopodium: False axis formed by joining up successive branches.

Puberulent: With very fine downy hairs.

Puberulous: Slightly hairy.

Pubescent: Covered with short, soft hairs.

Pulverulent: Dusted with fine powder.

Pulvinus: The swollen cushion like base of petiole.

Punctate: Dotted with depressions or with resinous glands.

Quincuncial: A type of aestivation, where out of five parts, two are exterior, two interior, and the fifth one having one margin exterior and other interior.

Raceme: An indefinte inflorescence in which the flowers are stalked and arranged on the long axis with the oldest flower near the base and the youngest near the top.

Racemose: Raceme-like.

Rachis: The axis of an inflorescence or of a compound leaf.

Radical: Arising from the root.

Radicle: The root of the embryo.

Ray floret: The small flowers or floret of capitulum situated near the periphery.

Receptacle: The part of the axis of a flower which supports other parts.

Reduplicate: A type of valvate aestivation where margins of each constituent project outwards.

Regma: A dry, schizocarpic fruit with elastically opening segments or cocci.

Regular flower: A flower which can be divided into two exactly equal halves by any vertical section passing through the centre.

Reniform: Kidney-shaped.

Repand: Undulate or wavy.

Replum: False partition wall developed by the extended placentae.

Reticulate: Net-like.

Retinaculum: The hook-like processes to which seeds remain attached.

Retuse: An obtuse leaf apex with a slight notch in the middle.

Revolute: A leaf with margins rolled lengthwise towards the lower side.

Rhachilla: The secondary axis in the inflorescence of grasses.

Rhizome: A thickened prostrate underground stem; usually horizontal.

Rootstock: Vertically growing rhizome.

Rostellum: A beak-like projection from the upper edge of the stigma in orchids.

Rotate: Wheel-shaped, usually referred to corolla.

Rotund: Somewhat circular in outline; usually applied to describe the shape of a leaf of waterlily, garden nasturtium, etc.

Rugose: Wrinkled. .

Rugulose: Slightly wrinkled.

Runcinate: Coarsely serrate to sharply incised with the teeth pointing towards the base.

Runner: A slender prostrate stem with long internodes, creeping on the ground, and rooting at the nodes.

Saccate: Gibbous.

Sagittate: Usually applied to the arrow-shaped leaf having basal lobes directed downwards.

Salver-shaped: Usually applied to corolla having a slender tube and an abruptly expanding limb; hypocrateriform.

Samara: A dry, indehiscent, 1 or 2-seeded, winged fruit, developing from a superior, bi or tri-carpellary ovary.

Samaroid: Winged fruits where the wings develop from dry, persitent sepals.

Saprophyte: The plant which lives on dead organic matter.

Scabrous: Pubescent.

Scaly: Scale-like.

Scape: The flowering shoot developed from underground stem.

Scapigerous: Scape-producing plant.

Scapose: Like a scape.

Scarious: Dry, thin, scale-like.

Sciophyte: Shade-loving plant.

Scorpioid: Scorpion-like; when the lateral branches develop on alternate sides forming a zigzag.

Scrambler: Weak plant which actually does not climb, but slowly grows over other bushes.

Scrub: A plant community dominated by shrubs or bushes.

Secund: Parts or organs directed to one side only.

Semiparasite: Partial parasite.

Sepal: The constituent of calyx.

Sepaloid: Like a sepal.

Septicidal: Usually applied to fruits where splitting takes place along the septa thus separating each loculus.

Septifragal: Usually applied to fruits where dehiscence is loculicidal or septicidal, but the valves fall off leaving the seeds attached to the central axis.

Septum: Partition.

Serrate: Margin with sharp teeth pointing forward.

Serrulate: Minutely serrate.

Sessile: Stalkless.

Setacious: Bristle-like.

Setose: Bristly.

Setulose: With minute bristles.

Sheath: The tubular basal portion of a leaf of a grass or sedge, which encircles the stem.

Sheathing: Usually referred to prominent leafbase which clasps and invests the stem.

Shrub: A plant which usually gives rise to a number of woody branches from the level of the soil forming a bush, in which the main trunk gets lost.

Sigmoid: Curved like 'S'.

Silicula: A short, broad and flat siliqua.

Siliqua: A dry, dehiscent, long, narrow, two chambered fruit developed from a bicarpellary pistil with two parietal placentae.

Simple fruit: A single fruit developed from the ovary of a flower with or without accessory parts.

Sinuate: With a deep wavy margin.

Sorosis: A multiple fruit developed from a spike or spadix.

Spadix: A spike with a fleshy axis and enclosed by one (sometimes more) large brightly coloured bract.

Spathe: Flat, broad, usually brightly coloured bract enveloping a spadix.

Spathellae: A speical name given to the spathes which separtately cover the branches of a compound spadix.

Spathulate or spatulate: Spatula-shaped leaf apex.

Spicate: Like a spike.

Spike: An indefinite, elongate inflorescence bearing sessile flowers.

Spikelets: A small spike; the unit of inflorescence of grasses and sedges.

Spine: Leaf or part of a leaf modified to a small, sharp, pointed, woody or hard body.

Spinose: Leaf-surface covered with prickles.

Spiral: Winding continually, usually applied to arrangement of leaves or floral organs.

Sporophyll: Spore-bearing leaf.

Sporophyte: Spore producing plant.

Spur: A tubular or sac-like projection, usually from the calyx or corolla, commonly producing nectar in its tip.

Squamose: Scaly or scale-like.

Squarrose: With minute scales.

Stamen: The pollen producing organ of a flower consisting of filament and anther; the unit of androecium.

Staminate: Bearing stamens; flowers which bear only stamens and no carpel is described by this term.

Staminode (*Staminodium*): A sterile or abortive stamen.

Standard (*Vexilum*): The broad outer petal in a papilionaceous flower.

Stellate: Star-shaped.

Stigma: The terminal end of the style, *i.e.*, the part that receives the pollen grains.

Stilt roots: Roots that grow obliquely downwards from near the base of the stem and provide additional support and anchorage.

Stipe: A stalk.

Stipel: Stipule-like appendages found on the two sides of the base of a leaflet.

Stipule: A pair of appendages present on two sides of a petiole at the base of some leaves.

Stolon: A slender lateral brance which originates from the base of the stem, bends down on or into the ground, and grows horizontally outwards for a shorter or longer distance.

Stoloniferous: Which produces or bears stolon.

Strap-shaped: Ligulate.

Style: The slender elongated projection of ovary, usually from top, and acting as the stalk of the stigma.

Subulate: Awl-shaped.

Sucker: A lateral branch of underground stem, but it grows obliquely upwards and gives rise to a leafy shoot or a new plant.

Sulcate: Grooved or furrowed.

Superior: Usually applied to an ovary which is situated above the point of attachment of perianth and stamens, or surrounded by a hypanthium that is not adnate to it.

Superficial: This term usually indicates origin from upper layers of tissues; also applied to the placentation when the placentae in a multilocular ovary is distributed all round the inner surface of the partition wall.

Suture: The line of union of two margins of one or more carpels.

Syconus: A multiple fruit developed from a hollow, pear-shaped, fleshy receptacle which encloses a number of minute, reduced, male and female flowers.

Synandrous: This a condition when two or more stamens are completely united by their filaments as well as anthers.

Syncarpous: Having carpels united.

Syngenesious: Stamens united by their anthers, often forming a cylinder around sytle.

Syngynia: When the ovaties or two adjacent flowers fuse while other parts remain free.

Taproot: The permanent root developed from the radicle via the stage of primary root.

Tassel: Apical panicles of maize on which the male flowers borne.

Taxonomy: Systematic botany, primarily concerned with the nomenclature and classification of plants.

Tegmen: Inner seed-coat.

Tentacles: Glandular hairs which secrete stickly fluid.

Ternate: In threes; trifoliate.

Testa: The outer and usually hard coat of a seed.

Tetradynamous: Having four long and two short stamens.

Tetramerous: When the number of floral members is four or multiple of four.

Thalamus: The suppressed swollen end of a flower-axis on which the floral parts, *viz.*, sepals, petals, stamens, and carpels are inserted.

Therophyte: Annual herb.

Thorn: A hard, often straight pointed structure develped usually through modification of axillary bud.

Thyrsus: Aspecial type of inflorescence having an indifinite main axis while secondary and other axes are of cymose nature.

Tomentose: Densely woolly with matted hairs.

Tomentulose: Delicately tomentose.

Trifoliate: A plamately comound leaf with three leaflets.

Trigonous: Three angled.

Truncate: A type of leaf apex, which appears as abruptly cut across or nearly so.

Tuber: The swollen end of a special underground branch of a stem, bearing scale-like leaves with buds (eyes) in their axils.

Tuberous: Tuber-like.

Twisted: Convolute, with parts rolled up in such a way that the outer part of each covers the inner part of the one in front of it, while in turn a part is covered by the one behind it.

Twiner: A plant that climbs by means of spirally coiling stems.

Umbellate: Of the from of an umbel.

Uncinate: Hooked.

Undulate: Wavy.

Unicostate: Having one prominent vein.

Unifoliate: A palmately compound leaf having only one leaflet.

Unipinnate: A pinnately compound leaf where the leaflets are directly borne on the midrib.

Urceolate: Urn-shaped hollow and contracted at the mouth.

Urticle: A small bladdery structure.

Valvate: A type of aestivation where the parts meet by their abrupt edges but not overlapping.

Valvular dehiscence: The whole or portions of the wall of anther open out like trap-doors releasing the pollens.

Veins: Rigid linear structures found in the leafblade, these form the fibro-vascular tissue system of the lamina.

Velutinous: Surface of a leaf is velvety, due to a coating of line, soft hairs.

Venation: The arrangement of veins of a leaf.

Vernation: Prefoliation, the mode or arrangement of leaves in the bud.

Vernicose: Shiny, as though varnished, leaf surface.

Verrucose: Surface covered with wart-like elevations.

Versatile anther: When filament is attached to merely a point on the back of the anther, so that the anther can swing freely.

Versicolor: Changing colour.

Verticillaster: A special type of inflorescence composed of a pair of opposed bichasial cymes bearing sessile or almost sessile flowers.

Verticillate phyllotaxy: Whorled phyllotaxy, more than two leaves at a node in a cricle around it.

Vexillary: Typical aestivation of the papilionaceous corolla where of the five petals, the posterior one almost covers two lateral petals, and the latter in turn nearly overlap the two anterior ones.

Vexillum: The posterior and usually the largest petal in the papilionaceous corolla.

Villose: Surface covered with long, soft and closely arranged hairs.

Viscid: Sticky.

Vitta: Tube in pericarp containing aromatic oil.

Vivipary: A kind of germination when seeds germinate inside the fruit while it is still on the parent tree and is nourished by it.

Viviparous: The plant in which vivipary takes place.

Whorl: A circle or cycle or ring of organs arranged around an axis, as the leaves in some stems, the organs of a flower.

Whorled phyllotaxy: Verticillate phyllotaxy.

Xeromorphic: Morphological character developed in xerophytes to facilitate them to adjust in the dry environment.

Xerophyte: The plant which can grow and subsist normally in dry localities like desert.

Zoophilous: Plants pollinated by animals.

Zygomorphic: A flower which can be divided into two similar halves by vertical section passing through one particular plane.

Appendix III
Conversion Factor

LENGTH

1 kilometre	=	10,000 metres = 0.621 mile = 1094 yards = 3281 feet.
1 metre	=	0.001 kilometre = 10 decimetres = 100 centimetres = 1000 millimetres = 1.0936 yards = 3.281 feet = 39.37 inches.
1 mile	=	8 furlong = 1760 yards = 5280 feet = 1.609 kilometres = 1609 metres.
1 yard	=	0.9144 metre = 9.144 decimetres = 91.44 centimetres = 914.4 millimetres = 3 feet = 36 inches = 2 hands (approx.) = 4 *bighats* (approx.).
1 foot	=	0.3048 metre = 3.048 decimetres = 30.48 centimetres = 0.33 yards = 12 inches.
1 inch	=	0.0254 metre = 0.254 decimetre = 2.54 centimetres = 0.083 foot.

AREA

1 hectare	=	100 ares = 10,000 square metres = 2.4711 acres = 0.8237 *bighas* = 0.4114 *cottahs.*
1 square mile	=	640 acres = 259 hectares.
1 square metre	=	10.765 square feet = 1550 square inches.

1 acre	=	0.4047 hectares = 4840 square yards = 43,560 square feet = 3 *bighas* (approx.) = 60 *cottahs* (approx.).
1 square foot	=	0.0929 square metres = 144 square inches.
1 square inch	=	6.452 square centimetres.

WEIGHT

1 ton	=	2240 lbs = 1000 kg.
1 lb	=	16 ounces = 0.4536 kg.
1 kg	=	2.2 lbs = 1000 g.
1 quintal	=	100 kg = 224 lbs.

Bibliography

ANON. *Cultivation of Medicinal Plants* (2001) National Medicinal Plant Board, Dept. of AYUSH, Ministry of Health & Family Welfare, Govt. of India.

ANON. *Hand Book of Agriculture* (2000) Indian Council of Agricultural Research, New Delhi.

ANON. *Hand Book of Horticulture* (2002) Indian Council of Agricultural Research, New Delhi.

ANON. *The Wealth of India* (1989) Vol. I to XI. Publications & Information Directorate, CSIR, New Delhi.

BENTHALL, A. P. (1984) *The trees of Calcutta and its neighbourhood.* Thacker Spink & Co. Ltd. London.

CHOPRA, R. N.; CHOPRA, I. C. & VARMA, B. S. (1969) *Supplement to Glossary of Indian Medicinal Plants.* Publications & Information Directorate, CSIR, New Delhi.

CHOPRA, R. N.; NAYAR, S. L. & CHOPRA, I. C. (1956) *Supplement to Glossary of Indian Medicinal Plants.* Publications & Information Directorate, CSIR, New Delhi.

DIETRICH BRANDIS (1921) *Indian Trees: An account of trees, shrubs, woody climbers, bamboos and palms, Indigenous or commonly cultivated in the British Indian Empire.* Constable and Company Ltd. London.

DRURY, C. H. (1978) *The Useful Plants of India.* Periodical Experts Book Agency, New Delhi 110 032.

FAROOQI, A. A. & SREERAMU, B. S. (2001) *Cultivation of Medicinal and Aromatic Crops.* Universities Press (India) Ltd. Hyderabad.

GUHA BAKSHI, D. N.; SEN SARMA, P. & PAL, D. C. (1999) *A Lexicon of Medicinal Plants in India.* Naya Prokash, Calcutta.

MUKHOPADHYAY, S. P.; BISWAS, K. & GHOSH A. (1973) *Bharatiya Vanoushadhy,* (*Vol. I to VI*) Calcutta University Press, Calcutta.

NAUTIYAL, M. C. & NAUTIYAL, B. P. (2004) *Agrotechniques for High Altitude Medicinal and Aromatic Plants.* Daya Publishing House. New Delhi.

PAL, D. C. & JAIN, S. K. (1998) *Tribal Medicine.* Naya Prokash, Calcutta.

SHARMA, R. (2004) *Agro Techniques of Medicinal Plants.* Daya Publishing House. New Delhi.

SUD, R. K. & KUMAR, S. (2004) *Herbs Culinary, Medicinal, Aromatic* (*Secrets & Human Happiness*).

Index